European Society for Medical Oncology

Handbook of Advanced Cancer Care

Edited by

Raphael Catane
Tel Hashomer, Israel

Nathan I Cherny
Jerusalem, Israel

Marianne Kloke
Essen, Germany

Stephan Tanneberger
Bologna, Italy

Dirk Schrijvers
Antwerp, Belgium

T0195315

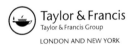

Taylor & Francis
Taylor & Francis Group
LONDON AND NEW YORK

© 2006 Taylor & Francis, an imprint of the Taylor & Francis Group
Taylor & Francis Group is the Academic Division of Infoma plc

First published in the United Kingdom in 2006
by Taylor & Francis, an imprint of the Taylor & Francis Group, 2 Park Square, Milton Park, Abingdon, Oxon, OX14 4RN

Tel.:   +44 (0) 20 7017 6000
Fax.:   +44 (0) 20 7017 6699
E-mail: info.medicine@tandf.co.uk
Website: http://www.tandf.co.uk/medicine

A CIP record for this book is available from the British Library.

Library of Congress Cataloging-in-Publication Data

Data available on application

ISBN 0-415-37530-4
ISBN 978-0-415-37530-6

Distributed in North and South America by

Taylor & Francis
2000 NW Corporate Blvd
Boca Raton, FL 33431, USA

Within Continental USA
Tel.: 800 272 7737; Fax.: 800 374 3401
Outside Continental USA
Tel.: 561 994 0555; Fax.: 561 361 6018
E-mail: orders@crcpress.com

Distributed in the rest of the world by
Thomson Publishing Services
Cheriton House
North Way
Andover, Hampshire SP10 5BE, UK
Tel.: +44 (0)1264 332424
E-mail: salesorder.tandf@thomsonpublishingservices.co.uk

Composition by Creative, Scotland

Printed and bound in Italy by Printer Trento

This publication has been supported by an unrestricted educational grant from
The European School of Onocology (ESO)

Contents

Appendix

Index

Foreword

It is my privilege to introduce this *Handbook of Advanced Cancer Care*, which belongs to a series of publications initiated by the European Society for Medical Oncology (ESMO). There is a great need, especially for medical oncologists, to have a comprehensive overview of the essential elements needed for the care of patients with advanced cancer. This handbook fulfills these requirements.

The *Handbook of Advanced Cancer Care* provides useful definitions and surveys of treatment principles. Excellent guidelines are provided for diagnostic procedures and therapies for various conditions associated with advanced cancer and its treatment. The chapters are written in a pedagogical manner with informative figures and tables and I believe this handbook will be of great value for all oncologists.

This handbook was written by experienced oncologists in their respective fields. I would like to convey my sincere thanks to all of them for their outstanding contribution. I am especially grateful to the editors, professors Raphael Catane, Nathan Cherny, Marianne Kloke, Stephan Tanneberger, and Dirk Schrijvers, for without their ceaseless efforts this excellent piece of work could not have been accomplished.

I am fully convinced that this ESMO *Handbook of Advanced Cancer Care* will serve as a reference guide for all oncologists and it is my sincere hope that you will find it useful and of great service.

Håkan Mellstedt, MD, Sweden
ESMO President

Treatment of advanced cancer

D Schrijvers
ZNA Middelheim, Belgium

1

Introduction

In most patients, cancer is diagnosed in an advanced stage. As a result of public awareness and screening programs, cancer diagnosis can be made at an earlier and more treatable stage, but many oncologists are still faced with patients with advanced disease.

It is important to know that, even in advanced cancer, anticancer treatment may improve survival and quality of life. Some tumors may be cured even in an advanced stage or quality of life may be improved or maintained with anticancer therapy. Supportive and palliative care should always be integrated in anticancer therapy, but the oncologist should be aware that even patients with advanced cancer benefit from anticancer therapy. Selection of patients as candidates for anticancer treatment is guided by sociocultural factors, the general condition of the patient, comorbidities, tumor type and stage, and available treatment modalities.

Curative anticancer treatment

Several tumor types may be treated with curative intent by surgery, radiotherapy, medication or a combination of these treatment modalities, even when the disease presents at an advanced stage (Table 1.1). Most childhood cancers and some of the cancers of adulthood and later ages are curable by combination therapy.

Palliative anticancer treatment

Several studies have compared the impact of both first- and second-line anticancer therapy with best supportive care in patients with advanced metastatic cancer. In patients with a good performance status, these treatments showed improved quality of life and improved survival (Table 1.2). However, for

Table 1.1 *Advanced-stage cancer that can be treated with curative intent*

Chemotherapy
■ Germ cell tumors of testis and ovary
■ Choriocarcinoma
■ Hodgkin's disease
■ High-grade non-Hodgkin's lymphoma
■ Acute lymphoblastic leukemia (children)
■ Acute myeloid leukemia
■ Small-cell lung cancer
Combination of chemotherapy and surgery
■ Rhabdomyosarcoma
■ Wilms' tumor
■ Osteosarcoma
■ Ewing sarcoma
■ Breast cancer
■ Epithelial ovarian cancer
■ Colorectal cancer
Combination of chemotherapy and radiotherapy
■ Cervical cancer
■ Anal cancer
■ Non-small cell lung cancer
■ Head and neck cancer
■ Lymphoma

several tumor types, there is a lack of randomized data comparing first- or second-line anticancr therapy with best supportive care, although many oncologists are in favor of treating these patients empirically if they have a good performance status (Table 1.3).

Treatment selection should be based on life expectancy and expected benefit for the patient (Figure 1.1).

Patients in good general condition should be offered the opportunity to participate in clinical trials.

Table 1.2. Improved quality of life and survival with anticancer therapy compared with best supportive care as shown in randomized trials

Tumor type	First-line therapy	Second-line therapy
Non-small cell lung cancer	Platinum-based	Docetaxel/pemetrexed
Colorectal cancer	5-Fluorouracil-based	Irinotecan
Pancreatic cancer	Gemcitabine	
Hormone-refractory prostate cancer	Mitoxantrone	
Gastric cancer	5-Fluorouracil-based	

Table 1.3. Empirical anticancer therapy suggested for therapy in advanced cancer in the absence of randomized studies with a best supportive care arm

Tumor type	First-line therapy	Second-line therapy
Adrenocortical carcinoma	Mitotane	
Head and neck cancer	Methotrexate Platinum-based	
Bladder cancer	Platinum-based	
Malignant glioma	Temozolomide	
Hormone-sensitive breast cancer	Tamoxifen Aromatase-inhibitors	Aromatase inhibitors
Hormone-refractory breast cancer	Anthracycline-based	Taxane-based
Hormone-sensitive prostate cancer	Castration	Antiandrogens
Gastrointestinal stromal tumor	Imatinib	
Endometrial cancer	Doxorubicin	
Renal cell cancer	Interleukin-2	
Malignant melanoma	Dacarbazine	
Ovarian cancer	Platinum-based	Taxane-based Topotecan Liposomal doxorubicin
Small-cell lung cancer	Platinum-based Anthracycline-based	
Thyroid cancer	Radioactive iodine	

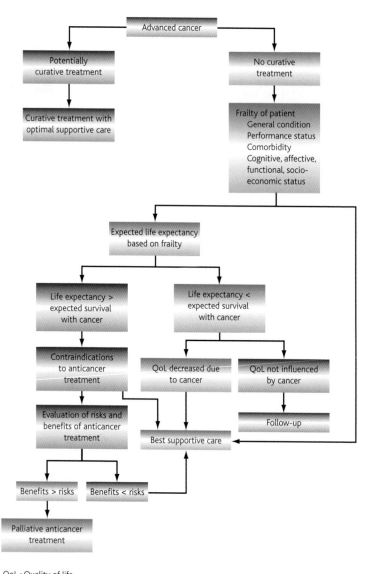

QoL : Quality of life

Figure 1.1 Approach to a patient with advanced cancer

Palliative care in advanced cancer

2

S Tanneberger
Fondazione ANT Italia, Italy

Introduction

In spite of much hope and some illusions, the cancer problem is far from being 'solved'. Global data show that cancer mortality is increasing worldwide. In the developing countries, cancer is one of the great challenges to health in this century.

The World Health Organization (WHO) predicts that by 2020 there will be about 10 million cancer deaths, of which 7–8 million will be accounted for by the developing countries, while the figure for the industrialized countries will remain unchanged at 2–3 million.

On the positive side, there will be a slight decrease in cancer mortality among younger people in the industrialized world, but this will be offset by the growing size of the aged population, with a high incidence rate of cancer in those aged over 75 years.

The age profile of cancer patients in the industrialized world is changing rapidly: in 2025, while 20–25% of the population will be older than 65 years, 50–60% of those dying of cancer will be older than 75 years. This means that oncologists will have to continue to deal with patients with a serious and life-threatening disease, many of whom will be terminal.

It would be wrong, both professionally and morally, to ignore these facts, and it is but proper that palliative oncology has developed rapidly in the last 20 years. Palliative medicine has a history of critical appraisal dating back to the start of the 'modern' hospice movement in the 1960s. However, based on the work of some pioneers, such as Dame Cecile Saunders in the United Kingdom and Vittorio Ventafridda and Franco Pannuti in Italy, palliative oncology has now gained recognition as a medical speciality within oncology, internal medicine and radiotherapy. Anesthesiology has made an enormous contribution to the treatment of pain in patients with advanced cancer.

By definition, palliative care starts when a cure is no longer possible. This is simple to say but not always easy to do. The tightrope walk between cure and palliation can become an ethical dilemma because the decision to palliate requires a change in treatment strategy. Palliative care in cancer is concerned with people who are likely to die in the near future from an uncontrolled malignancy. Palliative care is the quality of life rather than the length of life that is important. It is intended first of all to comfort and support those who are living with or dying from advanced cancer and their families.

A second problem is how to carry out palliative care. In spite of many discussions and recommendations, the practice of palliative care is not always in complete accordance with patients' needs and wishes. Sometimes, models for palliative care are developed that take into account economic, organizational and political aspects rather than the needs of patients. This should be avoided. Only the patient should be allowed to decide how he or she wishes to traverse, without losing dignity, the long and difficult path leading to the end of life ('eubiosia', as it has been called by Franco Pannuti).

The patient with advanced cancer

Every patient has individual feelings and needs. Sometimes, these are far from our expectations, organizational models and therapeutic approaches. Between patients living in developed and developing countries, there are differences with regard to not only the resources available for patients dying from cancer but also their experience of illness. Therefore, palliative care should be strictly patient-tailored. Nevertheless, the available clinical studies reveal some basic information about patients' emotions and their met and unmet needs, at least in the industrialized world (Tables 2.1 and 2.2). This information may guide the strategy and the best models for palliative care. Interestingly, the available data do not show very different emotions between those with early-stage cancer and those with advanced cancer.

Crucial points for palliative care in advanced cancer

Providing patients with palliative care is a challenge for the care-giving staff, from both the professional and the psychological points of view. Functional quality of life and symptom scores are significantly worse for 'last-minute' chemotherapy users than for nonusers. Among the organ- and symptom-specific problems, there are a few points to consider in any palliative care model for advanced cancer:

Table 2.1 What emotions do cancer patients have?

	Early cancer	Advanced cancer
To fight	55–60%	50–55%
Anxiety	15–20%	20–25%
Fatalism	15–20%	20–25%
Weakness	5–10%	5–10%
To ignore	1–2%	1–2%

Table 2.2 What are the fears of patients when life is ending?

Distance from their relatives and their home
Pain
Loss of personality
Loss of dignity
Emergency situations
Admission to the hospital

- Patients want not compassion but support and respect.
- In people with advanced cancer, not all observed symptoms are related to cancer.
- Prediction of an individual patient's life expectancy is correct in only about 30–40% of cases.
- Patients and their families often find it difficult to resist the promises of 'alternative cancer treatments' and need help.
- Diagnostic procedures without effective therapeutic consequences make no sense and can reduce the quality of a patient's life in such aspects as transport, cost or stress.
- Discontinuing anticancer treatment may be difficult and need more professionalism from the doctor than the decision to continue treatment.
- Communication means not only talking but also listening, feeling and touching.
- The patient has the right to know – but also the right not to know.
- The cost-benefit of palliative care should be understood as cost versus the dignity of life.
- Dignity of life depends very much on the place where palliative care is given.

What is the best place for palliative care in advanced cancer?

The best place is the place that offers the best quality of life to the patient. Seventy percent of advanced cancer patients want to be treated and to die at home. Therefore, it is preferable to bring palliative care to the patient and not the patient to palliative care. Unfortunately, this principle is not easy realizable in modern health-care systems.

For many patients, the hospital-at-home approach ensures comfort and dignity of life during the advanced and terminal phases of cancer. Hospital-at-home means that a full-time, professional palliative care team brings all that is necessary and available in a traditional hospital to the patient's home in order to ensure good palliative care. A hospital-at-home service should be a multidisciplinary and ideally a 24-hour service. Patients are visited at home, if required, every day and are in constant contact by telephone or other telecommunication.

The Bologna hospital-at-home service, which has 120 full-time physicians and 12 psychologists who take care daily of about 2500 advanced cancer patients, is an example of a successful hospital-at-home palliative care model. It has the advantage of starting care at an early phase of disease progression and can offer outpatient chemotherapy if necessary. Moreover, interventions such as ultrasound at home, radiography at home and blood transfusion and home enteral/parenteral nutrition are available. Costs are estimated at $100–200/day, which is less than the cost of a traditional hospital. The hospital-at-home has qualified and specialized staff who are further trained in palliative care. The problem is that this approach cannot be easily established in some traditional health-care systems.

Where the hospital-at-home approach is not possible, a general practitioner with special education in palliative care and enough time to use this education can offer palliative home care for advanced cancer patients. It is essential that there be close collaboration between the general practitioner, the oncologist, the pain specialist and the day-care center. Collaboration should also extend to the local network of social assistance and palliative nursing at home; this will help to guarantee the patient's dignity. Partnership and a spirit of collaboration between the different participants is essential in this multidisciplinary approach. This approach may challenge local health authorities to limit bureaucracy.

Although 70% of advanced cancer patients want to be at home at the end of life, home-care models are underdeveloped. They need powerful support from the medical community. The recent advances in communication technologies (telemedicine, flying televisits) offer enormous new possibilities for palliative care at home.

Discussions about home care often focus on costs, but such care can actually reduce the costs of health care. However, this reduction in cost sometimes means only the transfer of cost from the health-care system to the family. Research has consistently shown that family caregivers, too, often have a variety of unmet needs (their own ill health, insufficient skills to manage the patient's symptoms, inadequate support from health professionals and the financial burden of home care).

When the patient does not desire to stay at home or no caregiver is available, admission to a palliative care unit or a hospice can be an alternative. While hospice care remains an ideal model of care for cancer patients with terminal disease, the following obstacles in the clinical setting impede or prevent the otherwise appropriate referral of patients eligible for this type of end-of-life care:

■ a limited number of beds
■ high costs
■ issues of prognosis and communication
■ reimbursement.

Costs can be reduced by combining hospice care with an outpatient service (hospice-at-home). This has the advantage that the same doctor takes care of the patient during the outpatient and inpatient phases of terminal assistance.

Volunteers and volunteer organizations often support palliative care. This is an enormous contribution to the dignity of the patient's life and deserves the respect of every professional caregiver. Sometimes, the contributions of volunteers and nonprofit organizations are the only way to guarantee acceptable costs of palliative care.

Conclusion

Palliative care for advanced cancer patients has to be focused strictly on the control of symptoms and the psychological support of patients and their families. Patients should be protected from non-evidence-based overtreatment, which often reduces their quality of life. However, the decision to cure or to care can be difficult. Moreover, many patients want to continue to fight and to feel they are being 'treated'. The daily practice of palliative care should be tailored to the patient's needs, which we have to understand by careful exploration. Health-care professionals should encourage opportunities for carers to discuss their views of the ongoing needs of patients with advanced cancer.

Inclusion in clinical trials with protocols confirmed by an ethics committee is a reasonable approach for many advanced cancer patients. However, clinical trials of investigational treatments in patients with advanced cancer should pay appropriate attention to the patient's quality of life and supportive care issues.

Many palliative care patients prefer home care, and a majority of terminal patients want to die at home. For this reason, home care needs the greatest attention. However, the demographic situation makes it increasingly difficult to find family members who are willing to be caregivers at home. Therefore, parallel hospice organizations and palliative care units also deserve strong support. Only a well-organized network of specialized oncology, home-care and hospices/palliative care units can guarantee the fundamental human right of advanced cancer patients to live and die with dignity. Medical oncology should be the driver in establishing this network for palliative oncology.

Further reading

Ahmedzai SH: Supportive, palliative and terminal care. In: Cavalli F, Hansen H, Kaye SB (eds), Textbook of Medical Oncology, 2nd edn. London: Martin Dunitz, 2000: 665–89.

Higginson I: Clinical audit and organizational audit in palliative care. In: Hanks G (ed), Palliative Medicine: Problem Areas in Pain and Symptom Management. Cold Spring Harbor, NY: Cold Spring Harbor Laboratory Press, 1994.

Tanneberger S, Cavalli F, Pannuti F (eds): Cancer in Developing Countries. München: Zuckschwerdt Verlag, 2004.

Tanneberger S, Pannuti F, Mirri R et al: Hospital-at-home for advanced cancer patients within the framework of the Bologna Eubiosia project: an evaluation. Tumori 1998; 84: 376–82.

Twygross R: Symptom Management in Advanced Cancer. Oxford: Radcliff Medical Press, 1997.

Definition of palliative care

NI Cherny,
Shaare Zedek Medical Center, Israel

Introduction

There is much confusion about the definitions of palliative and supportive care. Some definitions have achieved wide acceptance, whereas other have been highly idiosyncratic. Oncologists have a unique perspective on the continuity of care and on the changing needs of cancer patients in different phases of the disease experience.

Goals of care

The goals of care set the context for clinical decision making and care planning. They can be summarized as three core elements: the prolongation of survival, the optimization of comfort and the optimization of function.

1. Prolongation of survival refers to the ability to cure, when possible, or to prolong survival, if this is desired.
2. Optimization of comfort is multidimensional, incorporating interventions to address physical, psychological, social and spiritual well-being. In many instances, the unit of care will include the patient and the family; consequentially, their comfort must be assessed and addressed according to need.
3. Optimization of function is, similarly, multidimensional. It includes physical, emotional and social function.

The relative priority of these goals is a continuum, and it changes in the course of disease progression. Typically, when patients present with early-stage disease, prolongation of survival takes precedence, and patients are commonly prepared to endure physical and emotional discomfort and sometimes impairment of function in pursuit of the main goal. At the other extreme of life – for example, the patient with debilitating dyspnea from advanced lung cancer – achieving comfort may be the main goal, even if the medication needed may impair cognition and communication and possibly shorten survival.

Phases of cancer

The diagnostic phase is characterized by unknown prognosis and undetermined relevant options.

Patients with potentially curable disease are not a uniform group, and the issues often differ among patients with a high, intermediate, low or very low likelihood of cure.

- *High likelihood of cure (>60%):* most patients are willing to undergo even difficult treatment programs. Refusal of treatment is distinctly uncommon.
- *Intermediate likelihood of cure (30–60%):* While most patients chose to undergo therapy, some patients, particularly at the lower end of the scale, may decline, particularly if treatment is particularly risky or onerous.
- *Low likelihood of cure (5–30%):* Patient decision making is much more heterogeneous, and is often influenced by treatment difficulty, and by impact of treatment on short and long-term comfort and function. What may be absolutely acceptable to some patients may be totally unacceptable (or even grotesque) to others.
- *Remote likelihood of cure (>0%, <5%):* Decision making in this setting is often difficult. If treatments are burdensome and/or risky, many patients choose to abstain. Some patients, however, seek aggressive and, sometimes mutilating or very high-risk therapies even if the likelihood of long-term benefit is very limited.

Patients with incurable disease are similarly heterogeneous. They can broadly be described as those who are either ambulatory or semiambulatory and for whom there is still the potential of improving the duration or quality of survival and those who are imminently confronting the prospect of death.

Among ambulatory or semiambulatory patients for whom treatment may improve duration or quality of survival, multiple factors affect decision making:

- Likelihood of response to treatment.
- Likelihood of clinical benefit: this includes both prolongation of survival and improvement of well-being.

- Likelihood of adverse effects and the potential seriousness of those effects on comfort and function.
- Physician bias: the oncologist's recommendations are a powerful determinant of patient decision making. Oncologists are not immune to bias: indeed, an oncologist's recommendation in this situation is fraught with bias. Like patients, oncologists' treatment practices can be described in a spectrum ranging from those who are very aggressive to those who are very conservative.
- Cultural and religious influences.
- Family influences.
- Economic considerations, particularly when treatments with potential benefit are extremely expensive or not covered by insurance.

Imminently dying patients are a subgroup with special needs. As death approaches, physical, emotional and spiritual problems become more common, more severe and more difficult to manage. Furthermore, the patient's impending death greatly affects the well-being and coping of family and friends.

Supportive, palliative and end-of-life care

Supportive care, palliative care and end-of-life care are related concepts. The multiplicity of these terms reflects the changing care needs of patients in different phases of their disease trajectory (Figure 3.1).

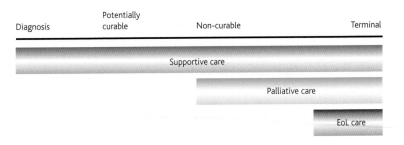

Figure 3.1 The relationship between supportive care, palliative care and end-of-life (EoL) care relative to the timeline of illness.

Supportive care

Supportive care aims to optimize the comfort, function and social support of patients and their families at all stages of the illness. This is a global term that is broadly applicable to all cancer patients. This care is characterized by:

■ optimal, stage-appropriate, anticancer care
■ prevention and management of side effects
■ optimal symptom control (physical and psychological)
■ optimal social support and family support
■ optimization of function.

Palliative care

Palliative care is the application of the principles of supportive care to the special conditions and needs of patients for whom cure is not possible. The emphasis of care is different because of the altered clinical and personal context of disease incurability.

In this context, palliative care incorporates a multidisciplinary approach focused on the patient's quality of life and coping as well as the coping and quality of life of the patient's family. This includes optimal symptom control (physical and psychological) and interventions to optimize coping, social support and family support. In many circumstances, anticancer care is an integral part of palliative interventions. In all cases, this must incorporate prevention and management of side effects.

Since many patients with potentially curable illness are ultimately found to be incurable, there is often no clear cutoff between potentially curative and noncurative treatment, and thus no clear cutoff in the transition from supportive to palliative care.

End-of-life care

End-of-life care is palliative care when death is imminent, emphasizing the special status of the patient and family associated with impending death. End-of-life care emphasizes optimal symptom control (physical and psychological) as well as social, psychological, spiritual and family support.

The interrelationship between these different care processes depends on the trajectory of the individual patient's disease (Figure 3.2).

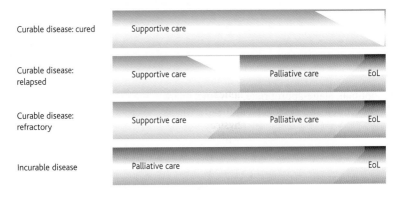

Curable disease: cured	Supportive care		
Curable disease: relapsed	Supportive care	Palliative care	EoL
Curable disease: refractory	Supportive care	Palliative care	EoL
Incurable disease	Palliative care		EoL

Figure 3.2 Transitions between supportive, palliative and end-of-life (EoL) care in four common disease trajectories

Infrastructural needs

The delivery of supportive and palliative care to cancer patients requires an appropriate medical nursing and paramedical infrastructure to address the special needs of patients and their families. It is the responsibility of medical oncologists to assess and evaluate physical and psychological symptoms of patients under their care and to ensure that these problems are adequately addressed.

The delivery of high-quality supportive and palliative care requires cooperation and coordination with physicians of other disciplines (including radiotherapy, surgery, rehabilitation, psycho-oncology, pain medicine and anesthesiology, and palliative medicine) as well as with paramedical clinicians (including nurses, social workers, psychologists, physical and occupational therapists, chaplains, and others).

Regarding end-of-life care for cancer patients, the European Society for Medical Oncology (ESMO) endorses the 'Core Principles for End-of-Life Care' (Table 3.1).

Table 3.1 The core principles of end-of-life care

Care at the end-of-life should:
1. Respect the dignity of both patient and caregivers
2. Be sensitive to and respectful of the patient's and family's wishes
3. Use the most appropriate measures that are consistent with patient choices
4. Make alleviation of pain and other physical symptoms a high priority
5. Recognize that good care for the dying person requires quality medical care, but also entails services that are family- and community-based to address psychological, social, and spiritual/religious problems
6. Offer continuity (patients should be able to continue to be cared for, if so desired, by their primary care and medical oncology providers)
7. Advocate access to therapies, that are reasonably expected to improve patients' quality of life and ensure that patients who choose alternative and nontraditional treatments are not abandoned
8. Provide access to palliative care and hospice care
9. Respect the patient's right to refuse treatment, as expressed by the patient or an authorized surrogate
10. Respect the physician's professional responsibility to discontinue some treatments when appropriate, with consideration for both patient and family preferences
11. Promote clinical and evidence-based research on providing care at the end of life

Source: Cassel CK, Foley, KM: Principles for Care of Patients at the End of Life: An Emerging Consensus Among the Specialties of Medicine. New York: Milbank Memorial Fund, 1999.

Further reading

Cherny NI, Catane R, Kosmidis P: ESMO takes a stand on supportive and palliative care. Ann Oncol 2003; 14: 1335–7.

Cherny NI: European Society of Medical Oncology (ESMO) joins the palliative care community. Palliat Med 2003; 17: 475–6.

How to integrate medical oncology and palliative medicine

4

M Maltoni
Morgagni-Pierantoni Hospital, Italy

D Tassinari
Infermi Hospital, Italy

In recent years, many authors have researched the integration of medical oncology and palliative care, identifying the union of these two disciplines as one of the main indexes for the definition of the quality of care. There are two important considerations within this context:

- The integration of primary cancer treatments (surgery, radiotherapy and medical oncology) and palliative care is necessary for physicians and caregivers to be able to guarantee the quality of care in the final stage of life.
- The need to integrate primary cancer treatments and palliative care is often disregarded due to the practice of administering chemotherapy up to the last stages of life, and of referring patients to palliative care programs only in the last days of life.

The coexistence of two opposite trends in clinical practice probably represents a transition period in which medical oncology and palliative care pass from being two different and independent fields of medical assistance for cancer patients (Figure 4.1) to a new approach in which both disciplines are integrated in a program of continuity of care (Figure 4.2).

However, the objective of continuity of care, besides being necessary to attain an adequate level of quality of care from diagnosis to the last part of life, is not easy to achieve because of the difficulty in organizing an integrated approach to patient care throughout all phases of the disease and also because of the lack of training and experience of medical oncologists in palliative care.

In recent years, the Task Force on Supportive and Palliative Care of the European Society of Medical Oncology (ESMO) has elaborated a program that can be divided into macroareas focusing on three priority fields of intervention (Table 4.1):

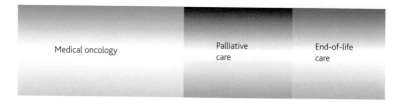

Figure 4.1 *The relationship between medical oncology and palliative care (traditional model)*

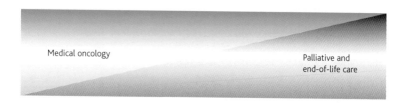

Figure 4.2 *The relationship between medical oncology and palliative care (innovative model). Characteristics: continuity of care; flexible primary care coordination (patient- or condition-determined); always goal-appropriate*

- an appropriate change of the oncologist's training and role, with the inclusion of adequate skills for the provision of supportive and palliative care
- training of oncologists in the treatment of the main syndromes of advanced or terminal disease
- palliative care services and oncological departments based on the modern concepts of continuity of care, favoring the integration of the two care dimensions in a single care concept.

A program promoting the integration of medical oncology and palliative care probably requires a multistep intervention in all three fields identified by the ESMO Task Force, and oncology departments or comprehensive cancer centers could represent the ideal locations to develop this approach. The ESMO Task Force has recently instituted a designation of excellence for centers integrating oncology and palliative care, where an integrated program could be documented and validated.

Table 4.1 *The three ESMO priority fields of intervention to improve continuity of care from diagnosis to the end of life*

The role of the oncologist in the provision of supportive and palliative care

Medical oncologists should play a role in the provision of palliative care:

- The medical oncologist must be skilled in the supportive and palliative care of patients with cancer and in end-of-life care
- The delivery of supportive and palliative care to cancer patients requires an appropriate medical nursing and paramedical infrastructure to address the special needs of these patients and their families
- The delivery of high-quality supportive and palliative care requires cooperation and coordination with physicians of other disciplines (including radiotherapy, surgery, rehabilitation, psycho-oncology, pain medicine and palliative medicine), as well as with paramedical clinicians

Supportive and palliative care training for medical oncologists

Medical oncologists must be skilled in supportive and palliative care of patients with advanced cancer. It follows that they must be skilled in:

- oncological management of advanced cancer
- communication with patients and their families
- management of the complications of advanced cancer
- evaluation and management of physical symptoms of cancer and cancer treatments
- evaluation and management of psychological and existential symptoms of cancer

They must also have:

- adequate knowledge of interdisciplinary care
- adequate knowledge of palliative care research
- adequate knowledge of ethical issues in the management of patients with cancer
- adequate knowledge of symptom control favoring factors and preventive strategies against burnout

Continued

Table 4.1 Continued

Minimal standards for the provision of supportive and palliative care by cancer centers
Minimal requirements of palliative care in a cancer center should include:
• periodic assessment of symptom burden during active treatment of cancer
• appropriate approach to resistant or intractable symptoms
• appropriate and prompt intervention against resistant or intractable symptoms
• adequate and prompt passage to palliative care services when the patient can no longer benefit from antitumor interventions
• social work and psychological care as part of the routine care
• adequate support in end-of-life care by a hospice or home-care service

Further reading

Cherny NI, Catane R: Attitudes of medical oncologists toward palliative care for patients with advanced and incurable cancer. Cancer 2003; 98: 2502–10.

Cherny NI, Catane R, Kosmidis P: ESMO takes a stand on supportive and palliative care. Ann Oncol 2003; 14: 1335–7.

Earle CC, Park ER, Lai B et al: Identifying potential indicators of the quality of end-of-life cancer care from administrative data. J Clin Oncol 2003; 21: 1133–38.

Maltoni M, Amadori D: Palliative medicine and medical oncology. Ann Oncol 2001; 12: 443–50.

www.esmo.org/WorkingGroup/designatedCenters.html

Surgery in advanced cancer

5

P Willemsen
ZNA Middelheim, Belgium

B Appeltans
Virga Jesse Hospital, Belgium

Introduction

Surgical intervention is an important aspect of the treatment of patients with advanced cancer, potentially enhancing quality of life. If complete resection can be achieved, surgery may even be curative. In selected patients with distant metastases confined to liver and lungs or even the brain, surgical resection of these lesions can be curative.

In many patients with advanced cancer, however, curative surgery is not achievable. If distant metastases are present, resection of an advanced primary cancer can be justified to treat severe symptoms such as bleeding, infection, pain or obstruction.

In a curative setting, surgical procedures and principles are clearly defined and well characterized. In a palliative setting, this is less clear. While 5-year survival, morbidity and mortality are of prime importance in the former situation, in the latter, quality of life, pain control and resolution of complaints are more pertinent therapeutic aims. Palliative care must select the treatment that will maximize quality of life and minimize complications. Whether or not to offer a surgical procedure to a patient with advanced cancer requires sound surgical judgment, as this decision can enormously affect the patient's final days. Up to now, there has been little evidence of the impact of palliative surgery.

Pain and symptom control are the main goals of palliative surgery, and good communication with the patient and family is essential to achieve the best results.

Patient selection

Selection of patients with advanced cancer as candidates for surgery is complex, and factors other than those normally considered in curative or nononcological surgery should be taken into account (Table 5.1). All of the

Table 5.1 *Patient selection for palliative surgery*

- Patient-dependent factors:
  - Chronological and biological age
  - Previous medical and surgical history
  - Patient's expectations
- Tumor-dependent factors:
  - Rapid/slow growing
  - Multiple or few metastases
- Surgeon-dependent factors:
  - Efficient surgeon
  - Good intraoperative appreciation of the situation
  - Communicative
- Family- and environment-dependent factors:
  - Realism about the procedure
- Postoperative do-not-resuscitate directives

following aspects need to be considered carefully before a palliative operation is performed:

- *Assess the patient.* The surgeon must estimate the patient's physiological age. What is the comorbidity and what is the expected impact of the surgical intervention on the patient? What is the patient expecting of a surgical intervention? Are the patient and family realistic about the surgical procedure?

- *Assess the symptoms.* A surgeon can do something about bleeding, infection, ulceration or obstruction, but surgical procedures are not going to alter fatigue, depression or anorexia. Therefore, to optimize the success of the surgical intervention, it is essential to recognize the chief complaints.

- *Assess the biology of the tumor.* Is the tumor rapidly or slowly growing? Are there few or multiple metastases? How is this going to interfere with the surgical intervention and the postoperative course?

- *Assess other treatment options.* What are the possible minimally invasive or radiological procedures? What are the noninvasive alternatives?

- *Assess previous treatments of the patient.* Has there been previous surgery? What type of chemotherapy has been used? Has the patient had radiotherapy? Previous treatments may influence the surgical procedure, and taking them into account can prevent serious complications.

- *Surgeons should assess themselves and the other surgeons involved.* Not only the surgical procedure is important. Intraoperative decisions may also be necessary: is the lesion causing the problem resectable or not, and at what cost? For successful palliation, it is good to have a compassionate surgeon. Before surgery, the goals of the procedure need to be clearly understood by both the patient and family and by the surgeon. This is the palliative triangle. Ideally, equal interactions between patient, family and surgeon will direct decision making, and in doing so, a patient-tailored decision can be made.
- *Assess the survival expectation.* What is a reasonable survival expectation? What are the severity of the presenting symptoms and the impact of the proposed procedure?
- *Do not talk patients into palliative procedures.* Before acceding to a patient's request to perform a procedure, a surgeon must be sure that the patient understands clearly what can and cannot be offered.
- When the decision is made to perform a surgical procedure in a palliative setting, it is important that directives for the postoperative period are clear. If there is a short expectation of life, a do-not-resuscitate (DNR) directive is critical and needs to be established beforehand. Obviously, the patient and family are involved in this decision.
- From all this, it becomes clear that patient selection for palliative surgery needs to be multidisciplinary and that the patient and family must be involved in this process.

Indications for surgery

A clear distinction between surgery with curative and palliative intent has to be made. In selected cases of advanced cancer, such as metastatic colorectal cancer confined solely to the liver or even liver and lung, a curative approach is still possible. In these cases, the extent of the procedure, the morbidity and the mortality and the chances for long-term survival must be discussed with the patient before a final decision is made.

In the palliative setting, treatment goals are different. If the patient is symptomatic, a surgical procedure can resolve bleeding, infection and abscess formation, ulceration, obstruction, or fractures. In selected cases, the symptoms caused by brain metastases can be surgically palliated. It is impossible to palliate an asymptomatic patient. The particular combination of local invasion and distant metastasis should tailor treatment strategies for palliative surgery in relation to complications.

The indications of palliative surgery are given in Table 5.2.

Table 5.2 *Indications for surgical intervention in a palliative setting*

Gastrointestinal tract obstruction
Bleeding
Infection and abscess formation
Skin ulceration
Fractures
Debulking of tumor causing severe symptoms

Palliative surgery in specific tumors
Abdomen
Gastrointestinal tumours
Upper gastrointestinal tumors
Gastric carcinoma

At diagnosis, gastric tumors are locally advanced in many patients, and it may take a few years before distant metastases develop. Therefore, it is worthwhile to aim for maximal debulking even in a palliative setting. However, extensive operations, including distal pancreatectomy and splenectomy, do not affect survival and they can create serious problems in postoperative management and may increase perioperative mortality significantly.

In the case of massive peritoneal spread and hepatic metastases, a simple bypass may resolve signs of obstruction, but removal of the primary tumor produces better palliation than a simple bypass.

The place of aggressive cytoreduction in combination with intraperitoneal hyperthermic chemotherapy in patients with peritoneal carcinomatosis secondary to gastric or colorectal cancer is still under investigation. In peritoneal carcinomatosis, this radical treatment will impair the quality of life, at least in the short term. However, these patients often present with distressing symptoms (obstruction, pain or dyspnea due to malignant ascites). The risk of such a procedure should be discussed with a patient willing to undergo this type of high-risk treatment without the possibility of cure but only a chance of increased survival time.

Pancreatic and periampullary carcinoma

In many patients who present with pancreatic carcinoma, curative treatment is not possible, either because of local unresectability or because of distant metastasis. Only 10–20% of patients with periampullary neoplasm are candidates for curative resection. The majority of patients cannot be treated with curative intent. In these patients, treatment must relieve the obstructive jaundice and the intolerable itching. Endoscopically placed bile-duct stents may resolve these symptoms.

The biliary–enteric bypass is a surgical option, and its effect usually lasts a lifetime for patients with unresectable periampullary cancer. However, this is a major intervention and may cause important complications, as observed in major intra-abdominal operations. This type of surgery may be performed laparoscopically (minimally invasive).

In some patients, the tumor causes gastric outlet obstruction or duodenal compression, and then surgical bypass of both the biliary system and the stomach is indicated.

An intraoperative chemical splanchniectomy can be performed for pain relief, especially in postprandial pain, although this procedure may be also be done by a percutaneous celiac axis block. Early involvement of anesthesiologists and pain therapists in the management of pain in patients with unresectable disease is highly recommended.

In otherwise fit and younger patients with locally advanced cancer, an R0 resection (Whipple or pancreatic tail resection), when technically feasible, results in good palliation.

Lower gastrointestinal tumors

Colorectal carcinoma

In advanced colorectal cancer with extensive liver metastases, intraperitoneal spread, local spread and involvement of adjacent organs, resection of the primary lesion is the better palliative option when there are signs of obstruction or anemia due to tumor bleeding. If resection of the primary lesion is technically not feasible, a bypass procedure can be performed. Resection of an obstructive tumor even in palliative circumstances has better results than bypass. In the unfit and frail patient, a simple diverting colostomy can resolve the symptoms of obstruction. These procedures can be performed by a classic open approach or by laparoscopy.

In most patients, gastrointestinal obstruction in advanced cancer is related to progressive disease. However, in some patients, the cause of obstruction is benign (e.g. simple adhesions) and might be easily treatable.

If a tumor perforates the abdominal wall and causes an abscess, this should be drained. Sometimes such an abscess is the presenting symptom of advanced colon cancer. Once the abscess is drained and the patient's condition improves, further diagnostic procedures can be carried out, and in some cases the tumor can be resected.

Thorax

Malignant pleural effusions

Surgery can play a role in the treatment of malignant effusions due to neoplastic disease. Pleural effusions can be voluminous and cause symptoms. Video-assisted thoracoscopy (VATS), drainage and talc pleurodesis can be used.

Malignant pericardial effusions

Sometimes, pericardial effusions occur in disseminated disease, and these can be treated either by percutaneous drainage or by creation of an internal pericardial window. This window can be made either subxiphoid through a small incision or minimally invasive through laparoscopy or as a VATS procedure.

Skeleton and extremities

Extremity sarcoma

The amputation rate for extremity sarcomas has fallen over the last 30 years. In the curative setting, surgery is mostly limb-sparing. However, in patients with local recurrence, nerve involvement, bone infiltration, pathological fracture or skin ulceration, amputation often is the only effective method of local palliation.

Bone metastasis and pathological fractures

The incidence of pathological fractures in patients with malignant disease is 1–2%, and 25% of all metastases to long bones progress to fractures. Pain, pathological fractures and hypercalcemia are the main causes of morbidity in patients with bone metastases. Bone metastases are an important cause of morbidity in patients with breast, lung, kidney or prostate cancer.

It is important to determine which patients with metastatic bone disease are at risk of developing a fracture. Surgical treatment of bone metastases aims at pain relief and preservation or restoration of function (Table 5.3).

Prophylactic fixation in patients with bone metastases clearly decreases morbidity compared with fixation of fractures. The difficulty lies in determin-

Table 5.3 *Surgery for bone metastases*

Indications for prophylactic fixation in bone metastasis	
Long bones:	Persisting/increasing pain despite completed radiotherapy
	Solitary, well-defined osteolytic lesion, >50% cortical circumference
	Proximal femur with fracture of the lesser trochanter
	Diffuse involvement of a long bone
Spine:	Spinal instability, bony compression of spinal cord, paraplegia
	Intractable pain, failure of conservative treatment
Contraindications for prophylactic fixation in bone metastasis	
Long bones:	Survival expectancy of <4 weeks
	Poor general condition, interfering with safe surgery

ing which patient requires prophylactic fixation. Many different criteria have been suggested, including the type of cancer, the size and the location of the metastatic lesion, pain due to the lesion, whether the lesion is osteolytic or osteoblastic, irradiation of the lesion, and the use of biomechanics to predict fracture. Prophylactic treatment is easier and less risky than treatment of an actual pathological fracture. Pathological fractures tend to heal slowly, and fractures in osteolytic metastases often end in nonunion of the lesion.

Emergency surgery is done for spinal metastases to preserve or save neurological function.

Central nervous system

Cerebral metastases

Quality of life is the main goal in the treatment of cerebral metastases. Corticosteroids in combination with surgery or radiotherapy are important to reduce cerebral edema, and reduction results in amelioration of the neurological condition. Symptoms such as hemiparesis, hemianopsia and speech disorders usually decrease or might even disappear. When patients require high doses of corticosteroids, or corticosteroids fail to relieve symptoms, surgery may be indicated. Surgical treatment is necessary when there is a need to diagnose metastatic cancer, especially in patients with an unknown primary tumor.

Side effects

Complications have a significant impact on palliative surgery: they interfere with the main goal of the palliative intervention and can interfere seriously with symptom control. Therefore it is important to try to minimize complications.

This starts with correctly assessing the patient and realistically setting the goals for palliative surgery. The appropriate surgical intervention should be chosen for the individual patient. All possible complications need to be discussed with the patient and their family in advance. Previous anticancer therapy should be inventoried. This influences the surgical options, and previous cancer chemotherapy may influence anesthetic management and postoperative recovery. Anemia, coagulation disorders, immunosuppression; pulmonary, liver, renal and cardiac toxicity, central nervous system complications, paraneoplastic syndromes, and metabolic complications influence anesthetic management and surgical outcome.

Peritoneal carcinomatosis is considered a 'hostile abdomen'. It can develop into a 'frozen' abdomen. In this situation, the surgeon has to know when to stop dissection before multiple enterotomies are created. Other forms of therapy need to be considered in this situation.

Several studies of surgery in malignant bowel obstruction reported an immediate postoperative mortality rate of 4–29%. The main goal, restoring oral feeding, was achieved in 42–85%.

Surgery may thus cause important side effects, and good and clear communication with the patient and relatives is imperative.

Conclusion

Surgical interventions have a place in the treatment of advanced cancer. It is very important that the patient and relatives are well informed about the type of surgery and what to expect from the surgical procedure. Similarly, the surgeon needs to know the patient's oncological and surgical history as well as the patient. This is important to make the right decisions before and during operation.

A multidisciplinary team approach is the best way to guarantee that everybody involved participates in the choice of the best treatment option for the individual patient.

Further reading

Cady B, Easson A, Aboulafia AJ, Ferson PF: Part 1. Surgical palliation of advanced illness – what's new, what's helpful. J Am Coll Surg 2005; 200: 115–27.

Cady B, Miner T, Morgentaler A: Part 2. Surgical palliation of advanced illness: what's new, what's helpful. J Am Coll Surg 2005; 200: 281–90.

Cady B, Barker F, Easson A et al: Part 3. Surgical palliation of advanced illness: what's new, what's helpful. J Am Coll Surg 2005; 200: 457–66.

McCahill LE: Methodology for scientific evaluation of palliative surgery. Surg Oncol Clin North Am 2004; 13: 413–27.

Miner TJ, Jaques DP, Shriver CD: A prospective evaluation of patients undergoing surgery for the palliation of an advanced malignancy. Ann Surg Oncol 2002; 9: 696–703.

6 Radiotherapy in advanced cancer

Y Lawrence, R Pfeffer
Sheba Medical Center, Israel

Introduction

Radiotherapy is useful in the palliation of several common problems in patients with advanced malignancy. These range from pain relief to the treatment of impending emergencies.

Radiotherapy uses ionizing radiation to kill cells. Palliative radiation is usually delivered externally by linear accelerators and cobalt machines. Shaped (conformal) radiotherapy beams and the choice of beam angles and energies help to minimize damage caused to normal surrounding tissues. For curative radiotherapy, the total dose of radiation is usually delivered by a number of smaller, daily fractions in order to reduce long-term side effects. In patients receiving palliative radiation, treatment may be shortened to a single fraction or to few fractions in order to improve patient comfort.

Radiotherapy is highly effective in dealing rapidly with anatomically localized problems, and if used judiciously it causes minimal side effects. Palliative radiation is underused, due to a combination of logistic difficulties, overstretched radiotherapy departments and patient/doctor misconceptions.

General principles of palliative radiotherapy

- Treatment should be:
  - based on the patient's symptoms, not imaging; asymptomatic metastases usually do not require palliation
  - as nontoxic as possible
  - planned in the context of the patient's overall disease status and performance status.
- It may require several days to achieve the palliative effect of radiation. Pharmacological treatments need to be continued during this period.
- For most patients, single, or short fractionation schedules are most appropriate.

- Treatment planning (often including computed tomography (CT) scanning) is required to define the target volume. It is important to avoid treating unnecessarily large volumes of normal tissue, which may produce toxicity.
- The treated area should be documented in case reirradiation is required.
- As in any other area of medicine, informed consent is the cornerstone of the decision. Dying patients should be able to refuse palliative treatments that others believe they should receive.
- When referring a patient to a radiotherapy service, it is necessary to include:
  - copy of original pathology
  - imaging studies (the radiographies and not just the report)
  - details of previous radiotherapy.

Bone metastases

The majority of patients referred for palliative radiotherapy suffer from painful bone metastases. Other symptoms associated with bone metastases include impaired mobility, pathological fractures, spinal cord compression and hypercalcemia.

Metastatic bone pain can be caused by:

- chemical stimulation of nociceptors
- pressure from the tumor or bone fragments on the periost
- direct pressure on nerves.

Rapid pain relief following a single fraction of radiation cannot be attributed to tumor shrinkage and may be due to reduced production of nociceptive chemicals. On the other hand, the component of metastatic bone pain due to pressure from bone fragments may require several weeks to heal after a course of radiotherapy.

Around one-third of patients receiving radiotherapy for bone metastases experience complete pain relief, and another third have significant reduction in pain. Several randomized studies have shown no significant difference in the degree, onset and duration of pain relief between multiple fractions (e.g. 10 fractions of 3 Gy each) and a single-fraction of 8–10 Gy. A Cochrane analysis concluded that single-fraction irradiation was as effective as multi-fraction irradiation, although more patients in the single-fraction arm (21.5% vs 7.4%) underwent retreatment with radiotherapy. The higher retreatment rate is not explained by less effective palliation, and it has been suggested that the main reason for this was that physicians were more willing to reirradiate after a single fraction than after a prolonged course of radiation. There is a small increase in fractures in patients treated with a single fraction (3% vs 1.7%).

Management principles of bone metastases

- A single fraction of 8–10 Gy is appropriate for most patients.
- Fractionated treatment (30 Gy in 10 fractions) should be considered when there is:
  - life expectancy of more than 6 months and few metastases
  - metastasis in a weight-supporting bone
  - spinal cord compression.
- Documentation of radiation fields is required (with simulation films or photography of skin-marked field boundaries), since up to 25% of patients require re-irradiation.
- Good margins are required; e.g. for vertebral metastases, add 1–2 vertebrae on each side of target lesion(s), and for limb lesions add 5 cm proximal and distal to the lesion.
- Nearby asymptomatic lesions may be included if toxicity will not be increased, especially if it is anticipated that they will soon become symptomatic.
- Minimize the volume of bowel/bladder in the radiotherapy field when irradiating the pelvis.
- Side effects of bone irradiation include:
  - bone-marrow suppression, dependent on the volume of marrow irradiated (important if chemotherapy is planned)
  - limb fibrosis and distal edema, which are preventable if the entire limb circumference is not irradiated.

Pathological fractures

- If the bone is already fractured (or there is an impending long-bone fracture), it is preferable to fixate the bone internally prior to irradiation, since radiation impairs callus formation. Radiation can be started within 48 hours.
- Candidates for operative fixation should have a life expectancy of more than 8 weeks and a reasonable cardiopulmonary function and performance status. Patients with pathological fractures who are not surgical candidates can achieve good pain relief from a single fraction of radiation.
- The fracture risk may be estimated by assessing the following recognized risk factors:

- size of metastasis: more than 50% bone diameter or more than 2.5 cm
- location: weight-bearing bones, particularly the peritrochanteric area of the femur, where even small areas of cortical involvement are dangerous
- type of lesion: radiolucent, osteolytic lesions more than osteoblastic lesions.

Other techniques of bone irradiation

Both wide-field (including hemibody) irradiation and strontium injection can achieve useful palliation for widespread bony disease. Contraindications include large extraosseous tissue masses and impending fractures.

Wide-field irradiation allows rapid relief of pain, starting within 48 hours and lasting for approximately 3 months. Previous tissue radiation doses must be taken into account. A dose of 8 Gy to the lower half of the body or 6 Gy to the upper half of the body resulted in good palliation for most patients. The use of bisphosphonates and radioactive strontium for patients with widespread bone metastases has led to a decrease in the use of hemibody irradiation.

Radioactive strontium is especially useful when external-beam radiation has been exhausted due to surrounding tissue tolerances. Onset of pain relief is usually within 10–20 days and may last up to 1 year. The technique is especially useful in breast and prostate cancer, although it should be used with care in patients heavily pretreated with chemotherapy due to the risk of prolonged pancytopenia.

Spinal cord compression

Spinal cord compression (SCC) is defined as compression of the dural sac and its contents (spinal cord and/or cauda equina) by an extradural tumor mass, with the appropriate clinical and radiological correlates. It often presents insidiously with back pain radiating in a belt-like fashion and may rapidly progress to overt neurological dysfunction, leading to incontinence and paralysis.

Median survival after diagnosis of SCC varies from 7 months in patients who are ambulatory at the end of treatment to 6 weeks for those with severe neurological impairment.

Management principles of SCC

■ Any cancer patient with radiating back pain should be suspected of having cord compression, especially if bone metastasis is present.
■ Early diagnosis before severe neurological symptoms develop is critical. Once paralysis develops, it is rarely reversible.

- Magnetic resonance imaging (MRI) is the optimal imaging modality. Imaging of the entire spinal cord is essential since 30% of patients have two or more points of cord compression.
- Corticosteroids are given for immediate relief until definitive treatment (radiotherapy or surgery) takes effect. An initial dose of 16–40 mg dexamethasone/day is often given.
- Radiotherapy is the primary treatment modality in the majority of patients.
- Typically, 30 Gy is delivered in 10 fractions over 2 weeks; shorter schedules, such as 10 Gy in a single fraction, are being investigated.
- Outcome after radiotherapy: 20% of patients improve neurologically, 30% stabilize and 50% deteriorate.
- Surgical decompression and debulking have a better outcome in selected patients. Relative indications for surgery include:
  - a single area of cord compression
  - good performance status prior to developing SCC
  - radio-resistant tumors (e.g. sarcoma, melanoma)
  - acute onset of paraplegia
  - radiological evidence of spinal instability, complete vertebral collapse or retropropulsion of bone fragments
  - requirement for pathological diagnosis.

Brain metastases

Symptoms attributable to brain metastases include headache, altered mental state, focal weakness and epileptic seizures. Symptoms usually develop over days and weeks, although a hemorrhage within a metastasis may cause sudden neurological deterioration. With the increased use of central nervous system (CNS) imaging, asymptomatic lesions are increasingly being diagnosed. MRI with high-dose gadolinium contrast is the most sensitive imaging tool for detecting brain metastases.

The rare case of a single brain metastasis in the absence of systemic disease may occasionally indicate curable disease and is an indication for resection or stereotactic radiosurgery. However, in the vast majority of patients, the primary aim of treatment is palliation of neurological symptoms, with prolongation of life being of secondary importance. It is justified to withhold brain irradiation in patients with extensive extracranial disease, poor performance status and short expected survival, since radiation is unlikely to prolong life and may produce more side effects than benefit.

The prognosis of patients with symptomatic brain metastases is 1–2 months without treatment, 2–3 months with corticosteroid therapy, and 3–12 months with whole-brain radiotherapy (WBRT).

Prognostic factors in patients with brain metastases include:
- primary tumor type
- age less than 65 years
- Karnofsky performance status ≥70
- controlled primary tumor.

Management principles of brain metastases

Corticosteroids

- Corticosteroids are the initial therapy for all patients. They decrease the inflammation and edema surrounding metastases. Symptoms may improve within 24 hours.
- A typical dose is 20 mg dexamethasone/day, which is slowly tapered.
- A histamine-receptor blocker or proton pump inhibitor is used to prevent gastric peptic ulceration.
- A good response to corticosteroids predicts a good response to brain irradiation.

Whole-brain radiotherapy (WBRT)

- WBRT is appropriate for the majority of patients with brain metastases.
- The standard dose is 30 Gy divided into 10 fractions.
- Short-term side effects include reversible alopecia, mild skin reaction, fatigue and sometimes ototoxicity.
- Long-term survivors of more than 1 year may suffer from varying degrees of dementia.
- Long-term local control is rarely achieved. However, 80% of the remaining life is with a stable or improved neurological condition.

High-dose single-fraction stereotactic radiation (radiosurgery)

Indications include:
- a single brain metastasis
- a small number of brain metastases unresponsive to WBRT (especially in radio-resistant tumors such as melanoma and renal cell carcinoma).

Surgical resection

- Indications are similar to those for stereotactic radiosurgery.
- There are no prospective trials comparing surgical resection and radiosurgery.
- Patients with a single highly symptomatic metastasis may especially benefit from the rapid relief provided by surgical resection.

Leptomeningeal carcinomatosis

The growth of tumor cells on the meninges is, except for acute leukemia, a preterminal event. Median survival is 1–4 months. Typical symptoms are disconnected neurological signs and symptoms combined with changes in mood and disposition. It is diagnosed by cerebrospinal fluid (CSF) cytology (three samples may be required) or meningeal enhancement on MRI scanning with gadolinium.

Treatment is with intrathecal chemotherapy with radiation directed to bulky, symptomatic disease as detected by MRI. The exact combination and schedule depends on local resources and the patient's prognosis and expectations.

Lung cancer

Inoperable non-small cell lung cancer (NSCLC) is a rapidly progressing, aggressive disease with limited treatment options. The close proximity of multiple critical structures within the mediastinal space underlies the complications experienced by these patients.

Either brachytherapy or external radiation can be used to palliate these patients. External radiation is less invasive and has a small survival advantage. Pain, cough and hemoptysis can be controlled in the majority of patients. However, vocal cord paralysis is rarely reversible.

Treatment planning of radiotherapy for NSCLC includes the following points:

- Encompass the whole tumor.
- Minimize the extralung volume.
- Include mediastinal nodes only if they are close to the primary tumor.
- It is preferable to use CT planning to reduce toxicities (esophagitis, pneumonitis or cardiotoxicity. However, it is not justified to delay the treatment in a symptomatic patient.
- Longer fractionation schedules have no advantage over shorter ones.

Superior vena cava syndrome

Large space-occupying lesions in the upper mediastial space may compress the superior vena cava, obstructing the return of blood to the heart. Frequently, secondary thrombosis forms within the vessel. Patients complain of dyspnea and facial swelling, and have distended neck veins. The most frequent cause is lung cancer, although lymphoma may cause up to 20% of cases. In most patients, a full workup and biopsy should be performed, although a rapidly worsening clinical picture may require urgent radiation, starting with large fractions (4 Gy). The total dose depends on the primary tumor (e.g. 30–40 Gy in lymphoma, 60–70 Gy in lung cancer). Over 75% of patients are successfully palliated with radiation.

In small-cell lung cancer, chemotherapy may be a more appropriate treatment.

Esophageal cancer

Esophageal cancer is a rapidly fatal cancer with a median survival of 9 months. Major complaints are odynophagia, dysphagia, cough and hemoptysis. Multiple modalities are available to palliate patients (surgery, brachytherapy, chemotherapy and endoscopically delivered treatments). The optimal role of each modality has not been defined. External-beam radiotherapy has the advantage of being noninvasive, with the ability to treat bulky disease outside the lumen. Seventy percent of patients may experience relief from dysphagia, although doses of over 50 Gy may be required.

Pelvic masses

Inoperable or recurrent pelvic tumors may cause severe pain (especially if the sacral plexus is involved) or obstruction of the urinary or gastrointestinal tract. If the disease is not metastatic, patients may survive for several years. CT planning is mandatory to evaluate the tumor volume and to enable the delivery of a large dose of radiation to achieve long-term palliation. Even if the pelvis has been previously irradiated (e.g. as adjuvant treatment for rectal cancer), it is usually possible to offer a further course of palliative treatment.

Bleeding due to cervical involvement may be palliated by hemostatic radiotherapy.

Further reading

Perez CA, Bray LW, Halperin EC et al: Principles and Practice of Radiation Oncology. Philadelphia: Lippincott Williams and Wilkins, 2004.

Sanghavi SN, Miranpuri SS, Chappell R et al: Radiosurgery for patients with brain metastases: a multi-institutional analysis, stratified by the RTOG recursive partitioning analysis method. Int J Radiat Oncol Biol Phys 2001; 51: 426–34.

Sundstrom S, Bremnes R, Aasebo U et al: Hypofractionated palliative radiotherapy (17 Gy per two fractions) in advanced non-small-cell lung carcinoma is comparable to standard fractionation for symptom control and survival: a national phase III trial. J Clin Oncol 2004; 22: 801–10.

van der Linden YM, Lok JJ, Steenland E et al: Single fraction radiotherapy is efficacious: a further analysis of the Dutch Bone Metastasis Study controlling for the influence of retreatment. Int J Radiat Oncol Biol Phys 2004; 59: 528–37.

Wai MS, Mike S, Ines H et al: Palliation of metastatic bone pain: single fraction versus multifraction radiotherapy – a systematic review of the randomised trials. Cochrane Database Syst Rev 2004; (2): CD004721.

Anticancer drug treatment

7

D Schrijvers, A Vandebroek
ZNA Middelheim, Belgium

Indications

The aim of anticancer drug treatment in patients with advanced cancer may be cure or palliation.Patients with advanced cancer in whom the aim of treatment is curative are infrequently seen, but cure is possible in certain hematological and solid tumors (Table 7.1). In most solid tumors, however, anticancer drug treatment aims to improve quality of life and disease-free, and sometimes overall, survival. In these patients, anticancer drug treatment should be considered only if quality of life may be improved and not impaired by the side effects of therapy.

Selection of patients for anticancer drug treatment

In patients with a tumor for which there is a potential curative treatment (Table 7.1), chemotherapy alone, or in combination with other treatment modalities, will be started even if the patient has a bad performance status and impaired organ function. Dose and schedule should be adapted according to organ function.

In all other patients, several factors should be considered before offering anticancer drug treatment (Figure 7.1).

Aim of the treatment

If cure is no longer an option, anticancer drug therapy should improve quality of life and may increase disease-free and overall survival. Treatment should not have a detrimental effect on quality of life. Most hormonal therapies used in the treatment of advanced breast and prostate cancer have a good toxicity/benefit profile, and they may be offered to these patients. Many chemotherapeutic regimens have a beneficial effect compared with best supportive care (Table 7.2), but at the cost of some toxicity. If the patient does not have any complaints due to cancer, and their life expectancy

Table 7.1 Advanced-stage cancer that can be treated with curative intent

Chemotherapy
• Germ cell tumors of testis and ovary
• Choriocarcinoma
• Hodgkin's disease
• High-grade non-Hodgkin's lymphoma
• Acute lymphoblastic leukemia (children)
• Acute myeloid leukemia
• Small-cell lung cancer
Combination of chemotherapy and surgery
• Rhabdomyosarcoma
• Wilms' tumor
• Osteosarcoma
• Ewing sarcoma
• Breast cancer
• Epithelial ovarian cancer
• Colorectal cancer
Combination of chemotherapy and radiotherapy
• Cervical cancer
• Anal cancer
• Non-small cell lung cancer
• Head and neck cancer
• Lymphoma

is not impaired by the malignancy, a period of follow-up without treatment is an option.

Patient-related factors

■ *Preference of the patient.* A patient should always give informed consent for anticancer drug treatment after information on tumor stage, treatment aim and side effects.

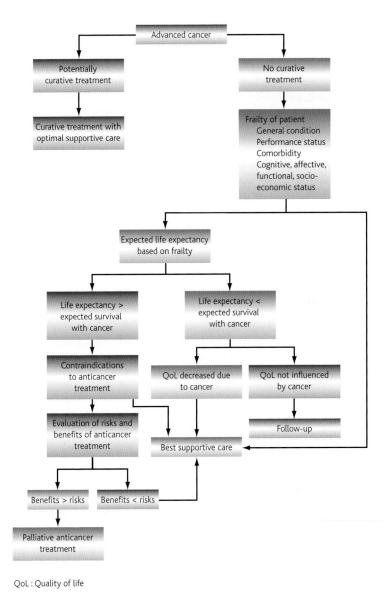

QoL : Quality of life

Figure 7.1 Approach to a patient with advanced cancer

Table 7.2 Improved quality of life and/or progression-free and/or overall survival with anticancer treatment compared with best supportive care in randomized trials

Tumor type	First-line therapy	Second-line therapy
Non-small cell lung cancer	Platinum-based Vinorelbine Gemcitabine Paclitaxel Docetaxel	Docetaxel Pemetrexed
Colorectal cancer	5-Fluorouracil-based	Irinotecan
Pancreatic cancer	Gemcitabine	
Hormone-refractory prostate cancer	Mitoxantrone	
Gastric cancer	5-Fluorouracil-based	

- *Age.* Many drug treatments are equally well tolerated by elderly and younger patients, and age as such should not be an important factor in a treatment decision.
- *Medical conditions*
  - *Malnutrition and weight loss.* Many patients with advanced cancer present with malnutrition and weight loss. Nutritional status may be evaluated by several self-administered questionnaires, and all patients should be weighed at their first visit and at each office visit thereafter. Patients should also have their height measured to calculate the body mass index, which should be between 22 and 27. Low serum albumin and cholesterol levels are prognostic factors for a higher chance of mortality. Serum albumin levels may decrease due to acute inflammation and stress.
  - *Performance status.* Most patients with a World Health Organization (WHO) performance status of more than 2 should not be treated with chemotherapy, as this may cause harm.
  - *Comorbidity.* Many cancer patients take drugs for other conditions, which may influence or be influenced by anticancer drugs (Table 7.3). Patients must be cautioned on the use of over-the-counter preparations and herbal medications, because there is limited knowledge on interaction between these drugs and anticancer drugs.
  - *Cognitive function.* The incidence of cognitive impairment increases with age and may influence informed consent and participation in

Table 7.3. Drug interactions of anticancer agents

Drug	Interaction
Asparaginase	Inhibits methotrexate; increases toxicity of vincristine; decreases synthesis of clotting factors
Bleomycin	Serum level decreased by digoxin, phenytoin
Capecitabine	Increases effect of warfarin; decreases metabolization of phenytoin due to interference with CYP2C9
Carboplatin	Decreases phenytoin level
Cisplatin	Other nephrotoxic drugs; decreases phenytoin level
Cyclophosphamide	Increases effect of warfarine; decreases digoxin level; metabolization increased by cytochrome P450 inducers
Cytarabine	Elimination decreased by nephrotoxic drugs
Docetaxel	Metabolization changed by drugs influencing CYP3A4
Etoposide	Increases effect of warfarin
Exemestane	Metabolization changed by drugs influencing CYP3A4
Fluorouracil	Activation inhibited by allopurinol
Gefitinib	Metabolization changed by drugs influencing CYP3A4
Imatinib	Metabolization changed by drugs influencing CYP3A4
Irinotecan	Metabolization changed by drugs influencing CYP3A4; increases effect of warfarin
Mercaptopurine	Bioavailability increased by allopurinol; decreases effect of warfarin
Methotrexate	Increased toxicity with nonsteroidal anti-inflammatory drugs, sulfonamides, trimethoprim
Paclitaxel	Metabolization changed by drugs influencing CYP3A4, clearance decreased when platinum compounds are given before
Procarbazine	Increased adverse effects with ethanol, sympathomimetics, tricyclic antidepressants, opiates, antihypertensive drugs
Tamoxifen	Potentiates effect of warfarin
Temozolomide	Clearance reduced by valproic acid

Continued

Table 7.3 Continued

Vinblastine	Metabolization changed by drugs influencing CYP3A4; decreases phenytoin level
Vincristine	Metabolization changed by drugs influencing CYP3A4; decreases digoxin and phenytoin level
Vinorelbine	Metabolization changed by drugs influencing CYP3A4

CYP..., cytochrome P450 isoenzymes. Inducers of cytochrome P450 include dexamethasone, carbamazepine, rifampicin, phenobarbital, phenytoin. Substrates of cytochrome P450 include simvastatin, cyclosporine, triazolobenzodiazepines, carbamazepine, dihydropyridine calcium channel blockers, fentanyl, warfarin.

treatment, palliative care and end-of-life discussions. Cognitive function should be assessed before initiating anticancer drug treatment.

  — *Affective status.* The depression rate in patients with advanced cancer ranges from 17% to 25% and is higher in women and in patients with poor performance and functional status. Risk factors that may predispose patients to develop depressive symptoms include social isolation, recent losses, tendency to pessimism, pain, history of alcohol and substance abuse, and socioeconomic pressure. Other causes of depressive mood should be excluded by determination of thyroid-stimulating hormone, vitamin B_{12}, calcium and liver function.

■ *Functional and environmental status.* Functional status is a predictor of response to cancer chemotherapy and an important measure of treatment toxicity. Functional status should be assessed before initiating therapy. Environmental assessment is important. Home hazards such as poor lighting, obtrusive electric and telephone cords, loose rugs, and absence of bathroom grab rails and stairway banisters can contribute to falls and physical disability. Environmental assessment also provides information on sanitary conditions, medication and nutrition.

■ *Economic status.* Cancer patients may be eligible for local or state benefits and for services for those with functional impairment. A social worker should help cancer patients determine their financial status and the benefits they may obtain.

■ *Social and spiritual status.* The social relationship structure of a cancer patient should be assessed by thorough history and enlisting a social worker. It is imperative that patients have a caregiver who is responsible for helping them when they are ill. Cancer patients also need emotional support and assistance from family and friends. Spirituality plays a large role in the care of cancer patients. Formal instruments have yet to be developed to assess spirituality, but asking patients whether religion and spirituality are important to them may provide insights to facilitate their care.

Drug-related factors

In patients with advanced cancer, pharmacokinetics may be altered, and this should be taken into account in drug selection.

- ■ *Absorption.* Most drugs are given intravenously, but oral formulations are becoming increasingly available. Absorption may be changed by gastrointestinal motility disorders, splanchnic blood flow, decreased secretion of digestive enzymes, and mucosal atrophy. Compliance of the patient with oral drug intake is of utmost importance.
- ■ *Distribution.* Volume of distribution is a function of body composition and the concentration of circulating plasma proteins (e.g. serum albumin and red blood cell concentration). A change in fat and intracellular water may lead to a change in the volume of distribution of polar drugs, influencing peak concentration and terminal half-life.
- ■ *Metabolism.* The liver is the main site of drug metabolization, and its function decreases with age. Metabolism occurs primarily by the cytochrome P450 microsomal system, which consists of a number of isoenzymes. Anticancer agents (e.g. cyclophosphamide, ifosfamide, paclitaxel, etoposide, teniposide, vincristine, vinblastine, busulfan and tamoxifen) are all substrates of the isoenzyme CYP3A4, which may be inhibited by a variety of commonly prescribed drugs. Another important way of metabolization is by conjugation.
- ■ *Excretion*
  - Renal excretion may be influenced by age, medication and other factors. Golmerular filtration rate should always be calculated by the Cockcroft–Gault formula. However, this formula is less accurate in populations with severe renal failure, and decreased muscle mass, as in the elderly. Decline in glomerular filtration rate translates into pharmacokinetic alterations of drugs or their active metabolites excreted by the kidneys. In cases of impaired renal function, chemotherapeutic agents primarily excreted by the kidney must be used with extreme caution, and dose modifications should be carried out (Table 7.4).
  - Hepatic excretion via bile is important for topoisomerase II inhibitors and taxanes. Impairment of liver function results in increased toxicity of these drugs, and dose reductions or adaption of schedules are indicated.

Table 7.4 Dose adjustments based on renal function

Drug	Creatinine clearance (ml/min)		
	≤ 60	≤45	≤ 30
Alkylating agents			
Melphalan	0.65	0.50	NR
Dacarbazine	0.80	0.75	0.70
Ifosfamide	0.80	0.75	0.70
Carboplatin	Calvert formula		
Cisplatin	0.70	0.60	NR
Oxaliplatin	No dose reduction if clearance > 20 ml/min		
Antimetabolites			
Hydroxyurea	0.85	0.80	0.75
Methotrexate	0.85	0.75	0.70
Fludarabine	0.80	0.75	0.65
Cytarabine	0.60	0.50	NR
Topoisomerase I inhibitors			
Topotecan	1.0	0.50	NR
Others			
Bleomycin	0.70	0.60	NR

NR, not reported.

Treatment of specific tumor types

In the case of a positive decision for drug treatment, patients should be offered participation in a clinical trial, especially if there is no standard treatment. If there is no clinical trial running or if the patient refuses participation, standard anticancer drug treatment in combination with best supportive care should be given (Tables 7.2 and 7.5). Standard treatment may vary according to national and local situations, but should be based on evidence-based or consensus treatment guidelines.

Side effects

Anticancer drug treatment always causes some side effects. Possible side effects should be discussed in advance with the patient, and points of

Table 7.5 *Empirical anticancer drug treatment suggested for treatment in patients with advanced solid cancer without randomized studies comparing treatment with best supportive care*

Tumor type	First-line therapy	Second-line therapy
Adrenocortical carcinoma	Mitotane	
Head and neck cancer	Methotrexate Platinum-based	
Bladder cancer	Platinum-based	
Malignant glioma	Temozolomide	
Hormone-sensitive breast cancer	Tamoxifen Aromatase-inhibitors	Aromatase-inhibitors
Hormone-refractory breast cancer	Anthracycline-based	Taxane-based
Hormone-sensitive prostate cancer	Castration	Antiandrogens
Gastrointestinal stromal tumor	Imatinib	
Endometrial cancer	Doxorubicin	
Renal cell cancer	Interleukin-2	
Malignant melanoma	Dacarbazine	
Ovarian cancer	Platinum-based	Taxane-based Topotecan Liposomal doxorubicin
Small-cell lung cancer	Platinum-based Anthracycline-based	
Testicular cancer	Platinum-based	
Thyroid cancer	Radioactive iodine	

attention should be addressed (e.g. neutropenic fever, bleeding due to thrombocytopenia). It is important to prevent these side effects or to start immediate treatment if they occur. Common side effects due to anticancer drug treatment and their prevention and treatment are given in Table 7.6.

Table 7.6 Common side effects of anticancer drugs

Side effect	Prevention	Treatment
Nausea and vomiting	5-HT$_3$ antagonist Dopamine antagonist Corticosteroids NK1 antagonists	5-HT$_3$ antagonist Dopamine antagonist Corticosteroids
Oral mucositis	Bland rinses (0.9% normal saline)	Topical anesthetics
Constipation	Laxatives	Laxatives
Diarrhea	Anticholinergics	Anticholinergics Octreotide
Anemia	Erythropoietin	Transfusion Erythropoietin
Thrombocytopenia		Transfusion
Neutropenia	G-CSF	G-CSF
Neutropenic fever	G-CSF	Broad-spectrum antibiotics G-CSF
Allergic reactions	Corticosteroids	
Asthenia	Exercise program	Adaption of lifestyle Exercise program

5-HT$_3$, serotonin (5-hydroxytryptamine) type 3 receptor; NK: neurokinin; G-CSF: granulocyte colony-stimulating factor.

Conclusion

Patients with advanced cancer should always be evaluated if they may benefit from anticancer drugs. Sometimes, a curative treatment can be offered, and every physician who deals with patients with advanced cancer should be able to identify these patients. In patients with incurable advanced cancer, the treatment decision should depend on the preference and clinical situation of the patient and the availability of a treatment that improves and maintains quality of life without causing severe side effects.

Gastrointestinal problems

D Tassinari
Infermi Hospital, Italy

M Maltoni
Morgagni-Pierantoni Hospital, Italy

Introduction

The clinical assessment and treatment of symptoms related to the gastrointestinal tract represent a significant problem in medical oncology and palliative care. Two questions must be considered:

- Is the gastrointestinal problem related to the tumor itself or is it secondary to the treatment of the tumor?
- Can the cause of the gastrointestinal problem be removed, or should one aim to provide symptom palliation only?

Moreover, several gastrointestinal symptoms may coexist in the same patient. It follows that a global approach should be applied in clinical practice.

Xerostomia and stomatitis
Prevalence

The incidence of xerostomia and stomatitis is 30–70% in patients treated with chemotherapy, radiotherapy or both, although they are only occasionally reported in patients with advanced cancer. Few data exist to assess their clinical relevance.

Etiology and differential diagnosis

Xerostomia and stomatitis are frequently related to iatrogenic causes. Two main conditions must be considered for differential diagnosis:

- those related to chemotherapy or radiotherapy (or both in concomitant treatments)
- those associated with supportive treatments (sedatives, prokinetics and anticholinergics).

A third situation, which may be iatrogenic, but may also be associated with the disease, is immunodeficiency-related stomatitis, frequently observed in patients with hematological tumors or HIV-related cancer, and in those on chronic treatment with corticosteroids.

Diagnostic procedures

A correct anamnesis and clinical evaluation are usually sufficient to assess the problem. Sometimes, when there is a suspicion of a viral or fungal superimposed infection, microbiological evaluation is useful for a differential diagnosis.

Etiological treatment

In all patients with chemotherapy- or radiotherapy-induced stomatitis and/or xerostomia, a critical analysis should be carried out of the side effects versus the benefit of treatment. Etiological strategies to improve the tolerability of treatments may include the use of chemo- and radioprotectants, a dose reduction or dose delay, drug modification (e.g. from 5-fluorouracil (5-FU) to capecitabine for the treatment of gastrointestinal tumors), or a change in the method of administration (e.g. from intravenous bolus to continuous infusion of 5-FU).

When stomatitis and xerostomia are secondary to supportive treatments, a different therapeutic approach is indicated, and a change in the class of drug responsible for the side effect is the most frequently used strategy.

When viral or fungal superimposed infection is strongly suspected or clinically documented, an etiological treatment should be added to supportive care.

Symptomatic treatment

The most common strategies used to combat the symptoms of stomatitis and xerostomia are correct oral hygiene, frequent mouth rinsing, citrus-based chewing gum or lozenges, or ice chips. The use of artificial saliva or pilocarpine can also be considered.

Dysphagia
Prevalence

Dysphagia is defined as difficulty in transferring liquids or solids from the mouth to the stomach. Although it is not a frequent symptom in metastatic cancer, occurring in 10–20% of patients referred to a hospice or palliative care service, it is frequently underestimated, especially when there is no clear clinical manifestation.

Etiology

Cancer-related dysphagia is frequently caused by mechanical obstruction. Tumors of the head and neck region or the esophagus, which are the main causes of dysphagia, are often asymptomatic in the early disease stages, but subsequently become clinically evident with pain or obstructive symptoms.

Dysphagia may also be iatrogenic as a consequence of surgery, radiotherapy or chemotherapy, with temporary or definitive damage to the anatomical structures of the upper gastrointestinal tract or to the intrinsic mechanisms of deglutition.

Two further causes of dysphagia that may be related to the tumor or to primary anticancer treatments are mycotic superinfection of oral, oropharyngeal or esophageal mucosa during primary or secondary leukopenia, and autonomic failure that alters normal pharyngo-esophageal peristalsis.

Diagnostic procedures and differential diagnosis

Anamnesis and clinical examination should be sufficient to diagnose dysphagia and to make a differential diagnosis. However, sometimes neither clinical information nor clinical examination of the mouth enables a definitive diagnosis, and further instrumental investigations (endoscopy, chest and mediastinal computed tomography (CT) scan, or functional examinations) are needed to identify the cause.

A differential diagnosis of the above-mentioned conditions is essential for a correct therapeutic approach, be it directed against the primary cause of the symptom or used as a supportive and palliative approach.

Etiological treatment

Surgery, radiotherapy or chemotherapy may be used as primary treatment for dysphagia when it is caused by a tumor obstructing the gastrointestinal tract. Anti-inflammatory or antimycotic treatment can be considered if dysphagia is secondary to an infection such as candidiasis. Sometimes the symptom may be a result of both tumor and primary treatment (chemo/radiotherapy), and the therapeutic approach must obviously take this into consideration.

Symptomatic treatment

In addition to primary treatment of the causes, supportive and palliative care of signs and symptoms that are related to dysphagia is fundamental to achieve the goals of primary treatment and to maintain quality of life.

Malnutrition represents one of the main clinical consequences of dysphagia, and nutritional support is important in the palliative approach. Enteral and parenteral nutrition are valid treatment options.

The aim of enteral nutrition is to overcome the obstacles favoring dysphagia. Parenteral nutrition, which is used when enteral nutrition is not feasible, usually requires a central venous catheter for an adequate supportive approach. Enteral nutrition is normally delivered through a nasogastric tube or enterostomy (gastric or duodenojejunal stomas). Generally, the choice in this type of alimentation is prognosis-driven, and the nasogastric tube is preferred in patients with a short life expectancy or in patients with transitory, reversible dysphagia. Enteral nutrition is preferred to parenteral nutrition because of its more physiological approach and in terms of quality of life.

Alternative procedures that favor natural alimentation (mainly in esophageal cancer) are the use of palliative endoscopy with laser or metallic stents that help to maintain a temporary normal alimentation.

Palliative medical treatment of dysphagia plays a minor role compared with primary treatment of the cause or with nutritional support. However, the use of prokinetics is considered useful when dysphagia is mainly due to autonomic nervous system failure.

Precautions

Patients with dysphagia should be carefully evaluated in both the diagnostic and the therapeutic phases. The patient should receive adequate support from the onset of symptoms to diagnosis, and treatment should take into account both the primary approach to the underlying causes and the support of the patient through all phases of primary treatment (if any).

Figure 8.1 illustrates a model of a diagnostic and supportive approach to dysphagia.

Nausea and vomiting
Prevalence

Nausea and vomiting are extremely frequent symptoms in patients with advanced or terminal cancer, occurring in approximately 60–70%. The

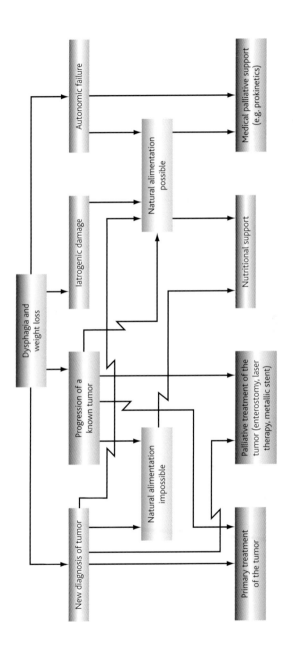

Figure 8.1 Diagnostic and therapeutic approach to dysphagia

53

clinical approach to assessment and treatment of the two different conditions is not yet evidence-based.

Etiology

Many factors induce nausea and vomiting in patients with advanced cancer, and more that one factor can contribute to their clinical occurrence (Table 8.1). It follows that the diagnostic procedures and the therapeutic approach should incorporate the coexistence of multiple factors favoring nausea and

Table 8.1 Causes of nausea/vomiting in cancer patients

Gastrointestinal causes
Gastric irritation
Gastric stasis
Upper gastrointestinal occlusion
Ascites
Hepatomegaly
Severe constipation
Metabolic causes
Hypercalcemia
Uremia
Infections
Sepsis
Candidal esophagitis
Drug-induced
Chemotherapy
Radiotherapy
Opiates
Digoxin
Antibiotics
Theophylline
Iron supplements
Central nervous system involvement
Raised intracranial pressure
Carcinomatous meningitis

vomiting. It also indicates the need for a heterogeneous strategy to control these distressing symptoms.

Diagnostic procedures and differential diagnosis

The first distinction should be made between cancer-related causes, which include occlusive and subocclusive syndromes, and iatrogenic causes, which include chemotherapy- or opiate-induced nausea and vomiting. Moreover, a central or peripheral mechanism may play a role in the pathogenesis, and although these pathogenetic pathways are usually analyzed separately, in clinical practice they often coexist in the same patient.

A complete and accurate anamnesis (including an accurate pharmacological anamnesis) and a clinical evaluation are the main steps to orient clinicians in their diagnostic approach.

Recent administration of chemotherapy or chronic treatment with opiates could lead to a 'toxicity hypothesis'.

Conversely, a clinical history of frequent subocclusive episodes and abdominal pain or clinical evidence of disorders in the intestinal tract would indicate an occlusive or subocclusive origin of the vomiting.

Another condition that may favor nausea is cancer-related anorexia, whose pathogenesis is associated with the simultaneous production of cytokines by the host's monocyte–macrophage system and by tumor cells. The diagnosis of and therapeutic approach to anorexia-related nausea are given in the section on the anorexia/cachexia syndrome in Chapter 9.

Radiological and endoscopic assessment of occlusive or subocclusive disease is indicated when an occlusion is suspected. This kind of approach may not be useful when the subocclusive status is known and the patient requires supportive care only.

Clinical assessment of nausea and vomiting in cancer and its follow-up in patients treated with etiological or supportive treatment is problematic. In addition to World Health Organization (WHO) criteria for the assessment of side effects during chemotherapy (which classifies vomiting into 5 grades by the number of episodes of vomiting), the clinical evaluation of nausea and vomiting in palliative care remains a partially solved problem, with no completely validated instruments for clinical assessment.

Etiological treatment

When a treatment is considered to cause nausea and vomiting, the patient should be reassessed to compare the side effects and benefit of the treatment responsible for these distressing symptoms.

■ Chemotherapy-induced nausea and vomiting seldom require a change in the choice of chemotherapeutic regimen, because of the efficacy of new categories of antiemetic drugs.

■ When nausea and vomiting are linked to chronic opiate treatment, the possibility of modifying either the opiate, the route of administration or both in so-called opioid rotation has to be considered.

When nausea and vomiting are secondary to occlusive or subocclusive conditions, a careful assessment of the patient is essential to identify an etiological approach. If a solitary blockage or an obstacle in the gastrointestinal tract can be documented, a surgical approach may be indicated. For all other conditions, which are more common in palliative care, an etiological treatment is usually not feasible, and only a symptomatic approach can be used.

Symptomatic treatment

Symptom control is the most frequent approach to nausea and vomiting in supportive and palliative care. Table 8.2 lists the most widely used antiemetic drugs for the treatment of nausea and vomiting.

Antiemetics, especially serotonin (5 hydroxytryptamine) type 3 receptor (5-HT$_3$) antagonists and corticosteroids, have radically modified the incidence of high-grade vomiting during chemotherapy, and guidelines have been published by different scientific organizations for their correct use.

In the case of gastrointestinal obstruction, the use of a venting nasogastric tube may be considered. Octreotide (1500 µg/24 hours subcutaneously) may be used to decrease gastrointestinal secretions and to reduce the frequency of vomiting.

Precautions

Although nausea and vomiting represent two of the most distressing gastrointestinal symptoms with different etiopathogenetic mechanisms, they can often be overcome by an accurate analysis of their causes (more than one condition can exist in the same patient), and by an adequately targeted treatment of the symptom.

Table 8.2. The most frequently used antiemetics in daily clinical practice

Class	Drugs	Indications
Prokinetics	Metoclopramide	Dysmotility Delayed gastric emptying Drug-induced nausea and vomiting
Corticosteroids	Dexamethasone	Acute and delayed chemotherapy-induced nausea and vomiting Subocclusive conditions Raised intracranial pressure
5-HT$_3$ antagonists	Ondansetron, granisetron, tropisetron	Chemotherapy-induced nausea and vomiting
Phenothiazines and butyrophenones	Promethazine, chlorpromazine, haloperidol	Symptomatic control of central and peripheral causes

Diarrhea and pseudodiarrhea

Prevalence

Diarrhea is not a frequent symptom in advanced or terminal cancer, occurring in 7–10% of patients admitted to a palliative care unit. However, it is a frequent side effect during chemotherapy or radiotherapy, often requiring a reduction in treatment dose intensity and worsening the quality of life.

Pseudodiarrhea may be the clinical manifestation of an occlusive or subocclusive condition.

Etiology

The conditions favoring diarrhea in cancer patients differ depending on the type of treatment. The main causes of diarrhea and pseudodiarrhea are shown in Table 8.3.

Diagnostic procedures and differential diagnosis

When diarrhea occurs in a cancer patient, a clinical distinction between an infectious and a toxic cause must be made to facilitate treatment.

The differential diagnosis between bacterial, viral or toxic diarrhea during chemotherapy or in a neutropenic patient is essential. Whenever there is

Table 8.3 Causes of diarrhea (and pseudodiarrhea) among cancer patients

Drugs	Laxatives
	Antibiotics
	Antacids
Chemotherapy	5-Fluorouracil
	Irinotecan
	Docetaxel
Radiotherapy	Pelvic radiotherapy
Intestinal obstruction	Fecal impaction with overflow (pseudodiarrhea)
Concurrent diseases	Inflammatory bowel disease
	Pancreatic cancer
	Biliary obstruction
	Fistula
	Short bowel
Neuroendocrine tumors	Carcinoid
	VIPoma

suspicion of infectious diarrhea, a fecal examination with stool cultures and tests for the etiopathogenetic microbial agent should be performed.

Moreover, when the cause of acute or chronic diarrhea in cancer patients is not clear, a laboratory fecal examination should be carried out to investigate the possibility of malabsorption.

In patients treated with antibiotics, *Clostridium difficile* toxins should be excluded.

Pseudodiarrhea due to fecal impaction with overflow must be kept in mind, especially in elderly, bedridden patients. Objective monitoring of the rectal ampulla by rectal examination with subsequent digital evacuation and laxative therapy should be carried out if necessary.

Etiological treatment

Drug-induced diarrhea often necessitates a modification in the choice or dosage, or both, of the etiological medication.

Infectious diarrhea usually requires adequate and prompt antibiotic treatment to avoid potentially serious consequences in neutropenic or debilitated patients. Antibiotics (amoxicillin–clavulanate or ciprofloxacin) are useful in the treatment of most bacterial diarrhea; *Clostridium difficile* diarrhea, which is often secondary to a protracted antibiotic treatment, should be treated with oral vancomycin or metronidazole.

Symptomatic treatment

All patients with diarrhea should be rehydrated. If the volume of diarrhea is copious and if the patient shows signs of dehydration, the risk of renal impairment or shock is high, and rehydration with electrolytes should be prompt.

Unfortunately, clinical quantification of the risk of dehydration during diarrhea does not exist, and clinical assessment of the patient remains the only means to identify the risk of a major dehydration syndrome.

In addition to the etiological approach, loperamide (the opiate of choice for its minimal intestinal absorption) or other opiates (morphine or codeine) can be used to reduce the number of bowel discharges.

Octreotide, a somatostatin analog, is indicated for intractable secretory diarrhea or diarrhea secondary to a neuroendocrine tumor.

Precautions

Diarrhea is a distressing symptom that can become serious or fatal without prompt and adequate treatment. An etiological approach should be accompanied by adequate supportive treatment with rehydration and pharmacological control of the number of bowel discharges.

Constipation
Prevalence

Constipation represents the most frequent symptom in cancer and noncancer patients, occurring in 45–60% of patients referred to palliative care services, and in approximately 40% of healthy people. It occurs in 90–95% of patients treated with opiates and does not show tolerance.

A distinction should be made between the personal concept of a normal evacuation rate, which could greatly differ from the real definition of constipation; an objective definition of constipation (fewer than three evacuations/week); and an occlusive status. It should be distinguished from anal tenesmus, which can often be confused with constipation by the patient, but which completely differs from an etiological and pathogenetic point of view. The lack of a clinical definition of constipation represents an obstacle in its clinical assessment, and even the concept of fewer than three evacuations/week, albeit supported by clinical rationale, cannot be considered conclusive from a clinical point of view and is often misinterpreted by patients and relatives.

Etiology

There are various causes of constipation in cancer patients, which can be classified into cancer-related causes, drug-related causes and comorbidity-related causes (Table 8.4).

Diagnostic procedures and differential diagnosis

The distinction between constipation and intestinal occlusion can be made on the basis of anamnesis and physical examination, or by radiological and endoscopic procedures (see the section below on acute and subacute malignant bowel obstruction) (Table 8.5). Physical and anamnestic data are usually sufficient to permit a diagnosis of constipation, whereas diagnostic procedures may be useful when an occlusive or subocclusive syndrome is suspected. Unfortunately, although the radiological findings of an occlusive condition are easily interpreted, borderline conditions often present unspecific radiological features, making a differential diagnosis difficult.

Etiological treatment

Sometimes, etiological treatment of drug-induced constipation can be adopted in cancer patients. In recent years, many authors have tried to find ways of reducing the incidence of constipation during chronic treatment with opiates, and changes in the opiates used or in the route of administration have been suggested as effective therapeutic approaches to this distressing side effect (opiate rotation). In particular, the use of transdermal fentanyl would seem to represent a valid alternative to oral morphine in patients with opiate-induced constipation. Similarly, the use of antipsychotics with low anticholinergic effect appears to reduce the risk of impaired gastrointestinal motility.

Symptomatic treatment

Laxatives are the symptomatic treatment of choice for constipation. However, when possible, every effort should be made to limit the conditions favoring constipation, such as bed rest, reduced motility, and low liquid and fiber intake. The choice of laxative treatment should be based on patient characteristics and clinical behavior (Table 8.6). Although no class of

Table 8.4 Frequent causes of constipation in patients with advanced or terminal cancer

Cancer-related conditions	Drugs-related conditions	Comorbidity-related conditions
Strictly related to the tumor:	Opiates	Diabetes
• Reduction of intestinal lumen	Anticholinergic agents:	Hypothyroidism
• External compression of gastrointestinal	• Spasmolytics	Electrolyte imbalance
lumen	• Phenothiazines	Large-bowel diverticula
• Neurological damage (central or	• Tricyclic antidepressants	Anal stenosis or anal rhagades
peripheral damage)	Antacids	Hemorrhoids
Consequences of neoplastic disease:	Diuretics	Colitis
• Starvation	Antihypertensives	
• Reduced alimentation	Antiepilepsy drugs	
• Dehydration	Vincristine and other	
• Asthenia	vinca alkaloids	
• Bed rest	Other chemotherapic agents	
• Delirium	5-HT$_3$ antagonists	
• Depressive conditions		

Table 8.5 *Differential diagnosis between constipation and bowel obstruction*

Constipation	Intestinal occlusion
• History of constipation, before and during the neoplastic disease • History of difficult defecation in the past • Correlation with the habits of the patient (alimentation, attitude to sports or physical exercise, emotional status) • Anorexia, nausea without vomiting (vomiting is extremely rare) • Atypical abdominal pain • Atypical radiological images	• Acute or subacute occurrence • Significant abdominal pain • Significant vomiting • Abdominal distention and lack of intestinal emissions • Typical radiological finding

Table 8.6 *Laxative medications*

Category	Mechanisms	Example
Bulking	Hydrophilic increase in fecal bulk	Dietary fiber, bran, psyllium
Osmotic wetting agents	Draw water into the intestine, promote peristalsis by mechanical distention	Lactulose Magnesium citrate Epsom salts Sorbitol Polyethylene glycols
Contact irritants/ stimulants	Alter water and electrolyte secretion. Stimulate colonic motility	Bisacodyl
Stool softener/ surfactant emollients	Promote mixing of fat and water, allowing fat to penetrate stool. Increased absorption of other laxatives	Docusate sodium
Lubrificants	Prevent absorption of water	Glycerin suppositories Paraffin oil
Enemas/suppositories	Local agents that distend colon, resulting in reflex evacuation	

laxatives is preferred to another for the different forms of constipation, a laxative ladder was recently proposed for the management or constipation. Furthermore, conditions increasing the risk of constipation, such as the start of treatment with opiates, should be adequately and prophylactically evaluated for prevention of constipation to avoid the occurrence or the worsening of this distressing symptom.

Acute and subacute malignant bowel obstruction

Prevalence

Bowel obstructions involving the abdomen are frequent in cancer patients. A tumor can cause bowel obstruction either directly, involving the gastrointestinal tract (as primary tumor or metastatic disease), or indirectly, by involvement of the peritoneal membrane. Although prevalence data vary with clinical context, malignant intestinal occlusions occur in approximately 10–50% of patients with abdominal tumors, in 4–28% of gastrointestinal tumors and in 5–50% of gynecological tumors (mainly ovarian cancer).

Etiology

All gastrointestinal tumors can cause bowel obstruction at the primary site. Moreover, they can lead to multiple sites of obstruction, either directly by involving different parts of the intestinal tract or indirectly by involving the peritoneal membrane. Ovarian cancers, which often give rise to acute or subacute intestinal obstruction in the course of their natural history (a common cause of death in ovarian cancer), usually affect the intestinal tract by peritoneal involvement, although direct metastatic involvement of the gastrointestinal tract is not uncommon.

Diagnostic procedures and differential diagnosis

The main differences between constipation and bowel obstruction are listed in Table 8.5. When clinical behavior suggests intestinal occlusion, a distinction in diagnostic and therapeutic approaches should be made between patients with and without a documented history of cancer. For patients with cancer, diagnosis of the site (or sites) of occlusion by clinical examination and radiological confirmation is sufficient for a therapeutic strategy, whereas in noncancer patients, diagnosis and staging of tumor are fundamental for correct management. Colon or gastric endoscopic evaluation and abdominal ultrasonography may also be required to define the primary condition causing the intestinal occlusion.

Etiological treatment

Surgical treatment of the primary tumor or the removal of a solitary relapse represent potential therapeutic approaches to bowel obstruction. In addition to surgery (which can be curative or palliative), radiotherapy and/or chemotherapy may also be indicated for an integrated palliative or curative etiological treatment. It is obvious that intestinal occlusions caused by chemotherapy-sensitive primary tumors may benefit from anticancer drug treatment more than those due to chemotherapy-resistant tumors. This highlights the importance of a careful selection of candidates for palliative chemotherapy.

Symptomatic treatment

The palliative treatment of intestinal occlusion is one of the most widely developed areas of palliative care, and many authors and various scientific organizations have established specific guidelines for the treatment of these patients. The European Association of Palliative Care guidelines for the treatment of intestinal occlusion are shown in Table 8.7. Surgical options and traditional medical management (nasogastric tube, massive hydration) have a modest role in the palliative approach to this problem, and medical treatments with haloperidol, morphine and anticholinergics or octreotide are more important for the treatment of these patients.

Moreover, intramural edema is successfully reduced by corticosteroids, whose efficacy is well established and whose mechanism of action seems to be related to an anti-inflammatory effect.

Similarly, the use of gastrographin, a hyperosmolar oral contrast medium, has been shown to be effective in reducing mural edema of the intestinal wall during intestinal occlusion.

Precautions

Bowel obstruction represents a problem for both patients with advanced cancer and noncancer patients. A preliminary distinction should be made between constipation and intestinal occlusion. Whenever there is a suspicion of intestinal occlusion, a further distinction should be made between patients who could benefit from primary treatment (especially surgery or chemotherapy) and those who require palliative care.

Table 8.7 *European Association for Palliative Care Guidelines for the treatment of inoperable intestinal occlusion*

Surgery. This does not represent the treatment of choice in the terminal phase of the disease due to the unfavorable cost–benefit ratio in this subset of patients
Self-expanding metallic stents. The use of stents is limited in these patients due to frequent occurrence of multiple stops
Nasogastric tube. The use of nasogastric tubes should be limited to draining abundant gastrointestinal secretions
Gastrostomy. Percutaneous endoscopic gastrostomy is a valid alternative to the nasogastric tube when the medical approach is inadequate to control the occlusive symptoms
Medical approach. This aims to reduce gastrointestinal secretions and vomiting and to control pain. The combination of anticholinergics, prokinetics and opiates represents the reference standard for the medical treatment of inoperable intestinal occlusions. Although octreotide would seem to be an interesting alternative to the above combination approach, as yet no definitive data exist to recommend its large-scale use in clinical practice
Artificial nutrition. This should be reserved for patients whose prognosis may be worsened by malnutrition. Adequate hydration should be reserved for all other (the majority) groups of patients

Anal tenesmus

Definition

Tenesmus is a painful spasm of the anal sphincter with an urgent need to defecate and involuntary straining, but little, if any, bowel movement.

Etiology

Anal tenesmus may have a cancer-related, infectious or iatrogenic origin. Tumor involvement of the rectum or perirectal tissue can cause tenesmus, as can some infectious agents, such as *Shigella* spp., *Campylobacter* spp. or *Clostridium difficile*, and iatrogenic sources, especially radiotherapy.

Diagnostic procedures and differential diagnosis

Both the diagnosis and differential diagnosis of tenesmus are clinical, although pelvic examination by endoscopic procedures, ultrasonography or magnetic resonance imaging (MRI) may be useful to define local damage.

When a patient presents with anal tenesmus, clinical investigations should aim at diagnosis of a new tumor or relapse, an infectious disorder, or an iatrogenic problem. Although differential diagnosis is important for a correct therapeutic approach, it is often difficult to distinguish between cancer relapse and radiotherapy-induced damage, and a biopsy is often needed to clarify the origin of this distressing symptom.

Etiological treatment

When tenesmus is due to a local tumor (anorectal, prostate or bladder cancer), a curative approach should be pursued whenever possible. When tenesmus is secondary to an infectious disease, appropriate antibiotic treatment should be given. When an etiological treatment is not feasible, symptomatic treatment should be given, especially in patients with advanced or terminal disease.

Symptomatic treatment

Radiotherapy or metallic stents play a role when surgery is not curative. Moreover, treatment with laxatives, opiates, and anti-inflammatory drugs or corticosteroids may be used for palliation. Although an etiological approach may be used in a number of specific conditions, a simultaneous palliative approach needs to be followed because of the variable response to specific treatments.

Anal tenesmus following radiotherapy usually resolves within 2–6 months, but in resistant cases, oral sulfasalazine, corticosteroids or sucralfate enemas can help to control the distressing symptoms.

Lumbar sympathectomy can also be used for a selected number of resistant conditions, but important side effects may limit this treatment approach.

The use of epidural opiates, local anesthetics and oral nifedipine has been described in this condition, but the modest efficacy restricts their use.

Ascites

Prevalence

Ascites is an accumulation of fluids in the abdomen that can be malignant (secondary to peritoneal carcinomatosis) or nonmalignant (hepatic cirrhosis). Although nonmalignant conditions are more frequent (80% of patients with ascites), the occurrence of ascites secondary to peritoneal carcinomatosis or to hepatic failure due to metastatic disease is not uncommon in clinical practice (approximately 10–15% of patients with ascites). Rare, nonneoplastic causes of ascites are heart failure (3%), tuberculosis (2%), nephropathies (1%) and pancreatic disease (1%).

Etiology

Many tumors cause peritoneal carcinomatosis and ascites, most frequently gastrointestinal and ovarian cancers. Moreover, some tumors cause hepatic failure due to massive metastatic involvement of the liver. Among nonmalignant causes of ascites, nonneoplastic hepatic failure, chronic heart failure and nephrotic syndrome are the main conditions that can be present in cancer patients.

Diagnostic procedures and differential diagnosis

The diagnosis of ascites in cancer patients is usually clinical. A modest quantity of ascites could be a sign of miliary peritoneal carcinomatosis, but this is an uncommon disease.

Confirmation of ascites is by ultrasonography. Cytological analysis is used when the origin of ascites is unknown: it permits the differential diagnosis between ascites secondary to peritoneal carcinomatosis or to hepatic failure.

Etiological treatment

Ascites secondary to chemotherapy-sensitive tumors may benefit from chemotherapy, whereas a more modest improvement has been observed in treating chemotherapy-resistant cancers. Both treatment-naive and pretreated patients with ovarian cancer show a reasonable response to chemotherapy, whereas a poorer response is generally obtained in patients treated for peritoneal carcinomatosis secondary to gastric or colon cancer. Encouraging results have been reported for treatment of chemotherapy-sensitive tumors involving the peritoneal membrane, but modest results have been obtained with chemotherapy for hepatic failure due to massive metastatic involvement of the liver.

Symptomatic treatment

The treatment of ascites is often palliative, and the aim is to improve ascites-related symptoms. There are three main approaches to the symptomatic treatment of ascites:

- the use of diuretics
- therapeutic paracentesis
- surgically derived procedures (although there is little evidence to support this approach in palliative care populations).

In particular, therapeutic paracentesis represents an easy, effective and safe approach that gives a rapid improvement of ascites-related symptoms and shortens the duration of hospitalization (from a mean of 30 to 10 days) without an increase in morbidity or mortality.

Clinical guidelines on paracentesis related to malignancy have been recently published, with particular attention to need of preliminary ultrasound examination, intravenous fluid provision and drainage time.

Gastrostoma management

Gastrostomy and jejunostomy are endoscopic, radiological or surgical procedures that may be used for palliation of gastrointestinal symptoms. These techniques can also be used for enteral nutritional support when oral nutrition is impossible, or for gastrointestinal decompression in occlusive or subocclusive conditions. In addition to the obvious indications for and limitations of the procedures for placing a gastrointestinal tube, careful follow-up of the stoma is needed. Table 8.8 describes the most important aspects that require monitoring. Acceptance and motivation of the patient and family, together with correct maintenance, are critically important for the successful management of gastrointestinal stomas in palliative care. Guidelines should be given for effective ostomy management, involving the establishment of an effective pouching system, modifications in dietary and fluid intake, and management of local complications.

Table 8.8 Suggestions for correct use and follow-up of gastrointestinal stoma

- Correct care of the tube exit site is essential
- Monitor the exit site of the tube for any peristomal redness, ulceration or drainage
- Flush, cap and connect the tube to the appropriate devices

Conclusion

Gastrointestinal symptom assessment and treatment represent one of the most important fields of palliative care for cancer patients. Such symptoms are frequently present in both advanced and terminal disease, and their burden is significant because of the negative impact on the quality of life of patients. The heterogeneity of clinical behavior is complemented by the heterogeneity of diagnostic and therapeutic approaches, and it is clear that a single approach cannot be adopted to a patient with one or more of these problems. In conclusion, quality of life remains the main outcome of the palliative treatment of gastrointestinal symptoms, and every effort should be made to guarantee an adequate palliative therapeutic approach to all of these symptoms in clinical practice.

Further reading

Bozzetti F, Amadori D, Bruera E et al: Guidelines on artificial nutrition versus hydration in terminal cancer patients. European Association for Palliative Care. Nutrition 1996; 12: 163–7.

Bruera E, Sala R, Rico MA et al: Effects of parenteral hydration in terminally ill cancer patients: a preliminary study. J Clin Oncol 2005; 23: 2366–71.

Cherny N, Ripamonti C, Pereira J et al: Strategies to manage the adverse effects of oral morphine: an evidence-based report. J Clin Oncol 2001; 19: 2542–54.

Cherny NI: Taking care of the terminally ill cancer patient: management of gastrointestinal symptoms in patients with advanced cancer. Ann Oncol 2004; 15 (Suppl 4): S205–13.

Doughty D: Principles of ostomy management in the oncology patient. J Support Oncol 2005; 3: 59–69.

Feuer DJ, Broadley KE: Corticosteroids for the resolution of malignant bowel obstruction in advanced gynaecological and gastrointestinal cancer. Cochrane Database Syst Rev 2000; (2): CD001219.

Glare P, Pereira G, Kristjanson LJ et al: Systematic review of the efficacy of antiemetics in the treatment of nausea in patients with far-advanced cancer. Support Care Cancer 2004; 12: 432–40.

Inui A: Cancer anorexia–cachexia syndrome: current issues in research and management. CA Cancer J Clin 2002; 52: 72–91.

Klaschik E, Nauck F, Ostgathe C: Constipation – modern laxative therapy. Support Care Cancer 2003; 11: 679–85.

Laviano A, Meguid MM, Rossi–Fanelli F: Cancer anorexia: clinical implications, pathogenesis and therapeutic strategies. Lancet Oncol 2003; 4: 686–94.

Maltoni M, Amadori D: Prognosis in advanced cancer. Hematol Oncol Clin North Am 2002; 16: 715–29.

Maltoni M, Nanni O, Scarpi E et al: High-dose progestins for the treatment of cancer anorexia–cachexia syndrome: a systematic review of randomised clinical trials. Ann Oncol 2001; 12: 289–300.

Regnard C: Dysphagia, dyspepsia and hiccup. In: Doyle D, Hanks G, Cherny NI, Calman K (eds), Oxford Textbook of Palliative Medicine, 3rd edn. Oxford: Oxford University Press, 2004: 468–83.

Ripamonti C, Twycross R, Baines M et al: Clinical-practice guidelines for the management of bowel obstruction in patients with end-stage cancer. Support Care Cancer 2001; 9: 223–33.

Stephenson J, Gilbert J: The development of clinical guidelines on paracentesis for ascites related to malignancy. Palliat Med 2002; 16: 213–18.

www.esmo.org/reference/referenceGuidelines/pdf/new_pdf/ESMO_13_NV.pdf

Alimentation/hydration

M Chasen
MUHC Oncology Program, Canada

N MacDonald
McGill University, Canada

Anorexia/cachexia syndrome
Introduction

The anorexia/cachexia syndrome is characterized by anorexia, weight loss (principally muscle loss), fatigue and often anemia. Cachexia is not simply due to decreased food intake or metabolic competition by the tumor. The syndrome appears to be primarily associated with aberrant inflammation (unbridled eicosanoid and cytokine production), which results in harmful changes in neuroendocrine-immune control.

A related problem is hypercatabolism, with wasteful body energy consumption and a loss of autonomic nervous system control. Manifestations of this include fatigue, cardiovascular alterations (postural hypotension, tachycardia) and gastrointestinal symptoms (constipation and early satiety).

Anorexia/cachexia arises from 'primary' systemic dysfunction induced by tumor presence. It is often associated with 'secondary' causes of wasting (see Table 9.1), which are often correctable. This condition is also seen in patients with other chronic diseases.

Weight loss is predictive of therapeutic response and survival. Different tumors produce different degrees of tissue loss; upper gastrointestinal and lung cancer patients commonly manifest it at first diagnosis. Gender influences cachexia; male lung cancer patients lose more weight than females.

Diagnosis and treatment

- It is important to differentiate cachexia from starvation (Table 9.2).
- One should identify and treat potentially correctable causes of secondary anorexia/cachexia (Table 9.1).
- If present, primary cachexia should be treated, in concert with good symptom control.

Table 9.1 Cachexia factor/treatment

Cachexia factor	Treatment
1. Psychological : • Anxiety • Depression	Psychotherapy Pharmacological
2. Eating problems: • Appetite • Disturbed taste	Dietitian
3. Oral: • Thrush • Dentures	Antifungal Oral moisteners
4. Swallowing difficulties	Esophageal dilation
5. Early satiety	Gastric stimulants
6. Nausea/vomiting	Various – related to cause
7. Fatigue/inability to sleep	Anxiolytics Antidepressants Exercise protocol
8. Motivation	Sleep protocol Exercise Methylphenidate
9. Pain	Analgesics Counseling
10. Metabolic: • Diabetes • Adrenal insufficiency • Hypogonadism • Thyroid insufficiency	As indicated

Anorexia

Prevalence

In systemic illness such as cancer, AIDS and chronic organ failure, anorexia (loss of appetite) is a very common symptom. Patients may lack the internal clock (hunger) that reminds them to eat, and this is often exacerbated by negative experiences of eating, fatigue and depression.

Table 9.2 *Starvation versus cachexia*

Starvation	Cachexia
1. Increased lipolysis	1. Increased lipolysis
2. Decreased proteolysis	2. Increased proteolysis
3. Reduced resting energy	3. Variable resting energy
4. Liver atrophy	4. Increased liver size
5. Reduced liver metabolism	5. Increased protein synthesis (acute phase)
6. Reduced glucose turnover	6. Increased glucose turnover

Etiology

Energy intake is mediated by the hypothalamus. Cancer-associated inflammation acts to inhibit the neurotransmitters stimulating appetite while enhancing the actions of those that reduce appetite and induce a sense of satiety. This neuromodulation appears to override appetite-stimulating hormones (e.g. ghrelin). Hypothalamic output in cancer patients may also contribute to adverse systemic changes, such as hypogonadism and hypercatabolism.

Approach

The assessment of the degree of anorexia/cachexia is important in planning any therapy. Simple questionnaires help to identify issues that must be resolved. Baseline use of the Edmonton Symptom Assessment System (ESAS) (see Appendix 1) and Patient Generated Symptom Global Assessment (PG-SGA), together with assessing function at home, is essential.

Approach to therapy

The loss of desire to eat affects social interaction with other family members, especially at mealtime. The overenthusiastic caregiver may place extra emphasis on the importance of eating and make mealtime difficult for the patient. Families will welcome a clear outline of possible approaches, which include the following:

Behavioral changes

■ increasing frequency of meals/snacks
■ diverting attention with social activity, such as television
■ planning ahead for low-energy days and taking advantage of 'best' mealtimes, such as breakfast

- avoiding cooking smells
- dietetics consultation
- liquid nutritional supplements
- recipe guides.

Medication

- *Glucocorticoids.* These are used to enhance appetite, although they are not consistently effective. Dexamethasone 3–6 mg/day or prednisolone 5 mg 3 x/day is effective in 60–80% of patients in the first few weeks of treatment. However no real additional effect beyond this period has been noted. Side effects are common and include acute delirium, glucose intolerance, irritation of the gastrointestinal tract, proximal myopathy (particularly with dexamethasone) and impaired immunity to *Candida* infection. A short course can be given to patients who have no contraindication, but if no improvement is seen after 1 week, therapy should be stopped. They are usually used later in the course of illness when efforts to maintain muscle are no longer paramount.
- *Progestational agents:*
  - Megestrol acetate (Megace®) increases appetite. The recommended dose is 480 mg/day × 24 days to establish efficacy. If it is not effective, therapy should be stopped. If appetite increases, the dose can be reduced to a lower one that remains therapeutic. Side effects include mild edema, impotence and, rarely, deep vein thrombosis. While megestrol is commonly used, an alternate progestational agent, medroxyprogesterone acetate, probably has similar effects. Progestational agents increase body mass (fat, not muscle) and can be catabolic with prolonged use. If used alone, they should be reserved for the time when appetite is paramount and muscle function is not.
  - Dronabinol (Marinol®) is a synthetic cannabinoid that increases appetite with little weight change. Dose is 2.5 mg two times a day. Side effects include dizziness and sedation.
  - Metoclopramide is a well-known antiemetic, but can be useful for patients with early satiety due in part to the increase in gastrointestinal transit time. Dose is 10 mg every 6–8 hours. Extrapyramidal side effects can occur.

Combined anorexia/cachexia therapy

Until recently, therapies concentrated mainly on the anorexia aspect of the anorexia/cachexia syndrome. The pendulum is swinging, and a high priority is now placed on maintenance of muscle and function. Therapies in this section include those that attempt to maintain lean body mass (muscle) although they may also have secondary, appetite-stimulating effects.

Agents now used in some programs

- *Amino acids.* Some trials suggest a net gain of lean body mass; they may have promise in combination therapy. Whey protein is a common source; some clinics use specific amino acids such as a mixture of glutamine, arginine and hydroxyl methylbutyrate.

- *Omega-3 fatty acids EPA (eicosapentaenoic acid and docosahexanoic acid) found in fish with dark flesh.* Supplementation can help maintain lean body mass in some patients with cancer, probably secondary to their anti-inflammatory effect.

- *Nonsteroidal anti-inflammatory drugs (NSAIDs).* Several European clinics have demonstrated their efficacy, alone or in combination therapies. Like omega-3 fatty acids, they modify unhelpful, tumor-associated inflammation. Studies have been published on ibuprofen, indomethacin and celecoxib. As many patients may be subject to 'polypharmacy' and otherwise sensitive to the adverse effects of NSAIDs, caution is advised.

- *Anabolic agents.* Many clinical studies have demonstrated that these agents can facilitate muscle growth. Testosterone levels are often reduced in patients with severe illness. Testosterone increases lean body mass, strength and weight in men with human immunodeficiency virus (HIV) infection and low testosterone. Some studies report improved function and quality of life. At present, it is reasonable to identify and treat hypogonadism with physiological testosterone doses. Use of higher doses remains a subject for research.

- *Exercise.* 'If you don't use it, you lose it'. Muscle function is dependent on muscle use. Within safe limits, patients should be encouraged to engage in mixed aerobic–resistance exercise programs.

- *Nutrition counseling.* This is particularly effective when used as part of a team approach including pharmacological stimuli and exercise guidance.

Compounds of interest not in clinical use for anorexia/cachexia, but as candidates for research

- *Angiotensin-converting enzyme (ACE) inhibitors.* The renin–angiotensin system is a master regulator of human physiology. Angiotensin II is activated by an enzyme that is blocked by ACE inhibitors. Activated angiotensin II increases the production of cytokines linked to inflammation.

- *Statins.* Studies demonstrate that statins have anti-inflammatory effects independent of their actions in cholesterol pathways. They consistently lower C-reactive protein (CRP). High CRP levels correlate with the presence of cachexia, tumor progression and survival.
- *Erythromycin and other 14-membered ring macrolide antibiotics with anti-inflammatory properties.* In two small Japanese trials, the use of clarithromycin correlated with both increased survival and improved body weight. Further studies are needed.
- *Creatine.* This is an important metabolite obtained through diet and synthesized de novo. The sports medicine literature proposes that muscles can be built up and enhanced; however, few crossover studies from sports medicine to disease-induced cachexia exist. Creatine is regarded as a safe supplement with minor adverse effects; however, patients with cancer and renal impairment who take creatine need careful monitoring.
- *Additional compounds of research interest:*
  - thalidomide
  - melatonin
  - β_2-agonists
  - tumor necrosis factor α (TNF-α) inhibitors
  - cytokine inhibitors
  - antioxidants
  - ghrelin
  - hypothalamic mediators – MC_4 antagonists
  - myostatin inhibitors.

Dehydration

Decreased oral intake is a complication of advanced cancer. This can result from many causes, such as profound anorexia, odynophagia, oral cavity lesions, dysphagia, bowel obstruction and cognitive impairment.

When oral intake is insufficient to hydrate the dying patient, some patients in a traditional hospital system may receive parenteral fluids, but others (and their doctors) may avoid their use.

The arguments *for* maintaining hydration in dying patients are as follows:

- Dying patients are more comfortable with parenteral hydration.
- Dehydration can cause confusion and enhance adverse drug effects.
- Oral hydration is given to dying patients who have thirst, so why not parenteral fluids?

- Parenteral hydration is a minimum standard of care.
- Withholding fluid to dying patients may result in withholding other therapies.

The arguments *against* hydration are as follows:

- Comatose patients do not experience symptom distress.
- Parenteral fluids may prolong the natural dying process.
- Less urine results in less need to void or for catheters.
- Without hydration, there is less gastrointestinal fluid, nausea and vomiting.
- Without hydration, there is less respiratory tract secretion.
- Without hydration, there is decreased edema and ascites.
- Dehydration may act as a natural anesthetic.
- Parenteral hydration is uncomfortable and limits mobility.
- Moistening and cleansing the mouth alleviates thirst.

Assessment

Assessment of hydration must take into consideration all symptoms, signs and laboratory findings. This is not a diagnosis to be based on a single symptom or sign. Assessment includes the following:

- intake
- output
- physical signs: dry mucous membranes, sweating, oliguria and postural hypotension
- presence of symptoms: cognitive failure, bedsores, nausea, fever, myoclonus and thirst
- laboratory findings: increased plasma proteins, hematocrit, blood urea nitrogen (BUN) and creatinine above baseline levels.

Therapy

Clinical studies suggest that terminally ill patients may achieve adequate hydration with smaller volumes than are needed by other patients due to:

- decreased body weight
- decreased clearance of free water.

Methods of fluid administration

The patient, family and multidisciplinary team must agree on rehydration (Table 9.3).

Table 9.3 Methods of fluid administration

Route of fluid administration	Indications
Intravenous	• If subcutaneous route is contraindicated • Intravenous line is otherwise needed
Subcutaneous (hypodermoclysis)	• With 150 units of hyaluronidase. Can be given as continuous infusion or bolus
Enteral	• For nutrition and hydration in patients with head and neck and esophageal cancer • Nasogastric tube versus gastrostomy tube

Fluid must contain:

■ electrolytes
■ potassium if there is diarrhea/fistula.

Opioids in hydration fluid should be avoided.

The volume is determined by the following formula:

minimum oral intake = daily urine output + 500 ml

Modes of alimentation
Nasogastric tubes

■ These are limited to patients with dysphagia from head and neck or esophageal cancers, who may benefit from nutrition/hydration.
■ There is no benefit for parenteral over enteral alimentation in patients with a functional bowel.
■ The enteral route is less expensive.
■ It can be done in a home-care setting.
■ Complications with nasogastric tubes include aspiration pneumonia, metabolic abnormalities, mechanical difficulties and nasal irritation.

Gastrostomy tubes

Percutaneous gastrostomy or jejunostomy can be performed under ultrasound guidance. They improve comfort and are useful for draining the intestinal tract in the case of inoperable bowel obstruction.

Protocol for care of gastrostomy feeding tube

■ The gastrostomy feeding tube is changed yearly, unless there is a specific need to do so more often.

■ Wash the hands with soap and water before handling the tube.

■ Gently clean around the tube twice daily with a disinfectant solution. Rotate and adjust the plastic bumper daily.

■ Do not apply a dressing around the tube, since this reduces the airflow and promotes infection.

■ Flush the tube after each feed with 150 ml tepid water. When the tube is not being used, still flush twice a day.

■ Report any redness, bleeding, pain or any significant change in the length of the tube.

Conclusion

When a patient with terminal cancer is severely dehydrated, the decision to rehydrate and feed should be made only after careful consideration of medical and psychosocial factors. Moral codes held by patient and family must be considered. If one is unsure of the role hydration will play, a short trial of hydration is appropriate. When it is considered appropriate, the subcutaneous route is preferred, as this will, in addition to being cheaper, also allow for home care.

Further reading

Bruera E, Fainsinger RL: Clinical management of cachexia and anorexia. In: Doyle D, Hanks G, MacDonald N (eds), Oxford Textbook of Palliative Medicine. Oxford: Oxford University Press, 1993: 330–7.

Fainsinger RL, Bruera E: The management of dehydration in terminally ill patients. J Palliat Care 1994; 10: 55–9.

MacDonald N, Easson AM, Mazurak VC et al: Understanding and managing cancer cachexia. J Am Coll Surg 2003L 197: 1143–61.

Steiner N, Bruera E: Methods of hydration in palliative care patients. Palliat Care 1998; 14: 26–13.

Walker P, Bruera E: Anorexia–cachexia syndrome. In: MacDonald N (ed),. Palliative Medicine: A Case-Based Manual. New York: Oxford University Press, 1998: 1–14.

10 Metabolic problems

D Colak, O Ozyilkan
Baskent University Faculty of Medicine, Turkey

Hypercalcemia

Prevalence

Hypercalcemia, the most common metabolic emergency in patients with cancer, occurs in up to 20–30% of patients with advanced cancer. The tumors that most commonly cause hypercalcemia are multiple myeloma, and breast, lung and renal cancers.

Pathogenesis

Tumors may cause hypercalcemia in two different ways: by direct invasion of the skeleton or by production of factors that stimulate osteoclastic activity. Among the latter, the most important is parathyroid-hormone-related protein (PTHrp). Others include osteoclastic activity factor, transforming growth factors, prostaglandin E, calcitriol, tumor necrosis factor, (TNF-α), 1,25-dihydroxyvitamin D and, very rarely, parathyroid hormone (PTH).

Diagnosis

In general, laboratories measure total serum calcium levels, which may be misleading, since fluctuations in albumin levels may affect measurement of total serum calcium levels. If there is any doubt about the validity of total serum calcium level, measurement of ionized calcium level is essential. There are also several formulas to adjust serum calcium levels to serum albumin concentrations such as the following:

$$\text{'corrected' calcium (mg/dl)} = \text{measured calcium (mg/dl)} - \text{serum albumin (g/dl)} + 4$$

In the case of hypercalcemia, all potential correctable causes should be ruled out. Total plasma calcium and ionized calcium; plasma albumin, phosphate and creatinine; total alkaline phosphatases; intact PTH; and urinary calcium, phosphate and creatinine levels should be determined.

The most common causes of hypercalcemia are primary hyperparathyroidism and cancer. In primary hyperparathyroidism, PTH levels are high or normal, whereas they are low–normal or low in hypercalcemia associated with cancer. Hypercalcemia in malignancy is usually obvious on clinical grounds. If there is suspicion, PTHrp measurement may be helpful.

Treatment

Treatment of hypercalcemia depends on the severity and the symptoms. Rate of occurrence, age and general status of the patient, concomitant diseases, and medication use are also important.

If possible, treatment of the underlying disease is most important, whereas severe and symptomatic hypercalcemia requires rapid and effective treatment.

- *General supportive measures.* These include encouragement of oral hydration and mobilization, decreased oral calcium intake, discontinuation of enteral or parenteral calcium supplements, elimination of drugs that may lead to hypercalcemia (e.g. thiazides, lithium, vitamin D and calcitriol), and discontinuation of sedatives (which may worsen neurological symptoms) and analgesics (which decrease renal blood flow).
- *Saline infusion.* The rate and amount of the saline infusion should be determined by the level of dehydration, the severity of hypercalcemia, and the cardiac and renal statuses of the patient.
- *Loop diuretics.* These block calcium reabsorption in the loop of Henle and make increased administration of saline possible by preventing hypervolemia. Since they may reinduce dehydration, their use should be restricted to patients who are fully rehydrated. Dosage administration depends on the patient's underlying renal function and hourly urine output. In general, 20–40 mg intravenous furosemide is administered initially, and subsequent doses are given when urine output is under 150–200 ml/hour.
- *Bisphosphonates.* These are the most effective and widely used agents in cancer-induced hypercalcemia. They inhibit osteoclastic bone resorption as well as calcitonin synthesis. The onset of action is 2–4 days, and the maximum effect occurs within 4–7 days. In severe cases, they should be used intravenously because of poor absorption from the gastrointestinal tract, but in mild cases, they may be used orally. The most commonly used bisphosphonates are pamidronate, zoledronic acid, clodronate and alendronate. The recommended dosage for pamidronate is 90 mg intravenously over 2 hours; and for zoledronic acid it is 4 mg intravenously over 15 minutes. A pooled analysis of two randomized, controlled clinical

trials showed that the efficacy of zoledronic acid is superior to that of pamidronate. Zoledronic acid also has the advantage of rapid and simpler administration, but it is more expensive. Both pamidronate and zoledronic acid have been reported to cause or exacerbate renal failure; serum creatinine should be monitored prior to each dose. In the case of unexplained renal dysfunction, both zoledronic acid and pamidronate should be discontinued until resolution of the renal dysfunction. In patients with pre-existing renal disease and creatinine values less than 3 mg/dl, no change in dosage, infusion time or interval is required.

■ *Calcitonin.* This has a rapid onset of action (2–4 hours), but the reductions in serum calcium are small and transient, and continued treatment is useless due to rapid development of tachyphylaxis. In the case of severe hypercalcemia, it can be added to provide an acute hypocalcemic effect. The recommended dosage is 4–8 U/kg salmon calcitonin intramuscularly or subcutaneously every 6–12 hours for 2–3 days.

■ *Other pharmacological agents.* Before the advent of bisphosphonates, drugs such as corticosteroids, mithramycin and gallium nitrate were used frequently. Today, they are used only when bisphosphonates are ineffective or contraindicated.

Endocrine paraneoplastic syndromes

Endocrine paraneoplastic syndromes result from inappropriate secretion of peptide hormones. These hormones are incompletely processed forms with reduced activity, and they are rarely suppressible. Endocrine paraneoplastic syndromes usually become evident only in patients with advanced malignancies, and successful treatment of the underlying malignancy leads to disappearance of the syndrome.

Syndrome of inappropriate antidiuretic hormone production (SIADH)
Prevalence

The syndrome of inappropriate antidiuretic hormone production (SIADH) is probably the second most common endocrine complication in patients with cancer. The most common malignancy associated with SIADH is small-cell lung cancer (SCLC), which comprises 75% of all cases; 3–15% of patients with SCLC develop the syndrome. Other tumor types causing SIADH are non-small cell lung cancer, neuroendocrine tumors, and squamous cell carcinoma of the head and neck.

Pathogenesis

The inappropriate secretion of antidiuretic hormone (ADH) impairs the ability to dilute the urine and leads to water intoxication with hypotonicity and hyponatremia.

Diagnosis

The diagnosis of SIADH is usually made on clinical grounds. Symptoms depend on the depth and the rate of development. Fatigue, anorexia, headache, altered mental status, seizures, coma and death may be seen.

The most common presenting sign of SIADH is hyponatremia, which is usually detected on routine laboratory evaluation in asymptomatic patients. The laboratory findings of SIADH include hyponatremia (Na < 135 mEq/l), hypo-osmolar plasma (< 280 mOsm/kg), and hyperosmolar and hypernatremic urine (urinary osmolality > 500 mOsm/kg; urinary Na > 20 mEq/l). In the differential diagnosis of hyponatremia, the evaluation of volume status is essential. Hyponatremia in SIADH is normovolemic. Other causes of normovolemic hyponatremia, such as hypothyroidism, renal dysfunction, Addison's disease and drugs causing hyponatremia (e.g. vasopressin, chlorpropamide, clofibrate, carbamazepine, vincristine, ifosfamide, nicotine and narcotics), should be ruled out.

Treatment

Symptomatology of patients and rapidity of onset of hyponatremia guide treatment strategy. Acute symptomatic hyponatremia in patients with a serum sodium level below 120 mmol/l requires immediate treatment. The treatment options are administration of hypertonic saline or concomitant administration of saline and furosemide. Since it may cause neurological damage and central pontine myelinolysis, hyponatremia should not be corrected too rapidly (not more than 1 mEq/l/h).

After correction of severe hyponatremia, and in asymptomatic patients, the goal of treatment is to balance the intake and clearance of free water. To achieve this, water restriction to 500–1000 ml/day is recommended. If water restriction alone is not enough, demeclocycline, which blocks the action of ADH, may be given at a dosage of 150–300 mg four times a day. Other medications reported to be beneficial are fludrocortisone, urea and lithium.

Ectopic adrenocorticotropic hormone (ACTH) syndrome

Prevalence

Ectopic adrenocorticotropic hormone (ACTH) syndrome occurs primarily in patients with SCLC (3–7% of all SCLC cases) and other tumors of neuroendocrine cell origin, and accounts for 10–20% of all Cushing's syndrome cases.

Pathogenesis

Tumors cause ectopic ACTH syndrome by releasing higher levels of ACTH precursors or producing intact ACTH.

In ectopic ACTH syndrome, cortisol and corticotropin levels are elevated, and the normal diurnal variation in their levels is lost. Hypokalemia and severe glucose intolerance may also be seen. Other signs and symptoms of ectopic ACTH syndrome include proximal myopathy, peripheral edema, muscle wasting, weight loss and hyperpigmentation. Because of the sudden onset, the classic signs and symptoms of Cushing's syndrome (such as truncal obesity, hypertension, moon face and buffalo hump) are not usually notable.

Diagnosis

The first step in diagnosis is to determine cortisol excess. Reasons for hypercortisolism include Cushing's disease, adrenal dysfunction, ectopic ACTH, and corticotropin-releasing hormone (CRH) overproduction. In adrenal dysfunction, plasma ACTH levels are low, whereas in other cases they are normal or high and tend to be higher in patients with ectopic ACTH syndrome.

The dexamethasone suppression test is also important in diagnosis. Low-dose dexamethasone suppresses cortisol production in healthy subjects, and high-dose dexamethasone suppresses production in Cushing's disease, but not in ectopic ACTH syndrome.

To test the adrenal–pituitary feedback loop, the metyrapone and CRH stimulation tests can be used. Metyrapone inhibits cortisol production in the adrenals and causes increased ACTH production in normal subjects and in subjects with Cushing's disease, whereas ectopic ACTH production is unaffected. In a patient with malignancy and signs and symptoms of ectopic ACTH syndrome, nonsuppressible hypercorticolism is usually sufficient to make the diagnosis. For definitive diagnosis, inferior petrosal sinus sampling with administration of ovine CRH is necessary.

Treatment

As far as possible, treatment of ectopic ACTH syndrome is by resection of the tumor; however, this is rarely possible. In surgically unresectable cases, the treatment of choice is cytotoxic chemotherapy for the primary malignancy, which is combined with medical or surgical adrenalectomy. Especially in surgical adrenalectomy, to avoid adrenal insufficiency, a lifelong replacement therapy of glucocorticoids and mineralocorticoids is also needed. In medical adrenalectomy, the choice of drugs is aminoglutethimide, metyrapone and ketoconazole. Octreotide and mifepristone may also be used.

Hypocalcemia

Etiology

Hypocalcemia in malignancy is associated with lytic bone metastases, malignancies that secrete calcitonin (primarily in medullary carcinoma of thyroid gland, and rarely in other malignancies such as breast, colorectal and lung cancers), hypomagnesemia (inadequate oral intake or prolonged parenteral alimentation), hyperphosphatemia (tumor lysis syndrome) and overconsumption of calcium by the tumor. Decreased serum albumin levels may lead to 'false' hypocalcemia, and in cases of hypoalbuminemia, serum calcium levels should be verified by serum albumin levels or ionized calcium levels should be measured.

Diagnosis

Most patients are asymptomatic; however, fatigue, muscular weakness, neuromuscular irritability, confusion, muscle cramps and sometimes tetany, laryngeal stridor or convulsions may be seen.

Treatment

Treatment strategies depend on the underlying cause and on the severity of symptoms. In mild cases, oral calcium supplementation can be given, but in severe cases, calcium infusion should be administered.

Further reading

Arnold SM, Lieberman FS, Foon KA: Paraneoplastic syndromes. In: De Vita VT Jr, Hellman S, Rosenberg SA (eds), Cancer: Principles and Practice of Oncology, 7th edn. Philadelphia: Lippincott: 2005: 2189–2211.

Drüeke TB, Lacour B: Disorders of calcium, phosphate, and magnesium metabolism. In: Johnson RJ, Feehally J (eds), Comprehensive Clinical Nephrology, 2nd edn. New York: Elsevier, 2003: 123–40.

Hillner BE, Ingle JN, Chlebowski RT et al: American Society of Clinical Oncology 2003 update on the role of bisphosphonates and bone health issues in women with breast cancer. J Clin Oncol 2003; 21: 4042–57 (erratum 2004: 22: 351).

Parikh C, Kumar S, Berl T: Disorders of water metabolism. In: Johnson RJ, Feehally J (eds), Comprehensive Clinical Nephrology, 2nd edn. New York: Elsevier, 2003: 87–108.

Stewart AF: Clinical practice. Hypercalcemia associated with cancer. N Engl J Med 2005; 352: 373–9.

Respiratory problems

AC Grigorescu, M Marian
Institute of Oncology, Romania

Introduction

Millions of people worldwide suffer from respiratory symptoms resulting from lung cancer and pulmonary metastases. Respiratory symptoms such as cough and dyspnea are common in patients with advanced and incurable disease, giving rise to varying degrees of respiratory distress that adversely affect quality of life. Other major respiratory problems are death rales, acute suffocation and hemoptysis.

In recent years, there have been significant advances in the palliation of respiratory symptoms, leading to practical ways of providing relief in hospices and hospitals and at home.

Dyspnea
Prevalence

Dyspnea involves the unpleasant sensation of being unable to breathe easily, and it causes anxiety in both patients and their caregivers. Dyspnea is a subjective experience of difficult, labored and uncomfortable breathing, which may be described as shortness of breath, a smothered feeling, inability to get enough air or suffocation. Dyspnea is one of the most commonly reported symptoms in lung cancer, with an incidence of 15% at diagnosis and 65% in the final stages of the disease.

The prevalence of dyspnea varies with the site of the primary malignancy, the stage of disease, and other factors. During the last days of life, dyspnea is seen more frequently. In patients with non-small cell lung cancer (NSCLC) and small cell lung cancer (SCLC), the prevalence is as high as 85%.

Etiology

The causes of dyspnea in advanced cancer are multiple (Table 11.1) and they can be classified according to:

- local or systemic causes
- relationship with tumor (malignant, paramalignant, nonmalignant)
- physiological impairment:
  - lung function pattern (obstructive, restrictive or mixed)
  - oxygen saturation (hypoxic or nonhypoxic)

The identification of causes of dyspnea guides their treatment. However, treatment options are often limited by the performance status and poor prognosis of the patient.

Diagnosis

The severity of dyspnea is not predictable by respiratory function tests, which in most patients are not useful in assessing the need for treatment or monitoring. The subjective nature of dyspnea requires an assessment based on the patient's description. Patients often have several different underlying factors that lead to the development of dyspnea.

Evaluation of the underlying causes relies on medical history, detailed physical examination and carefully selected investigations. Medical history should include smoking habits, occupational exposure, drug history, past anticancer treatment, concomitant medical illness, associated respiratory symptoms and pattern of dyspnea. Tachypnea (rapid breathing) often accompanies dyspnea. If panic and anxiety are present, they lead to a central increase in the rate of breathing, which further increases the feeling of breathlessness and anxiety. A prospective study of 100 terminally ill cancer patients (49 with lung cancer) showed that dyspnea, measured on a visual analog scale, was significantly associated with anxiety ($P=0.001$). Increased anxiety has been associated with more severe dyspnea in cancer patients. One study of 120 patients with stages I–IV lung cancer showed no difference in dyspnea in relation to cancer stage, cell type or performance status. However, pain and anxiety scores were higher in patients with high dyspnea scores.

Investigations should be carefully selected to guide specific treatment. The most important investigations are hemoglobin level, oxygen saturation (oximetry, a noninvasive method to identify hypoxic patients) and chest radiography, which may be informative in defining specific syndromes.

Dyspnea evaluation scales

There are scales measuring multiple symptoms including dyspnea and scales for measuring dyspnea alone.

Table 11.1 Causes and symptoms of dyspnea

Mechanism	Malignant causes of dyspnea	Associated symptoms
Upper airway obstruction	Intraluminal tumor Extrinsic compression by tumor or lymph nodes	Wheezing, stridor
Acute superior vena cava obstruction	Compressed or invaded by tumor Secondary thrombosis	Facial swelling, moderate venous distention, symptoms and signs of raised intracranial pressure
Chronic superior vena cava obstruction	Lung cancer 75% Lymphoma 15% Other cancers 10%	Markedly distended veins of the upper chest and arms
Bronchial obstruction	Tumor causing loss of lung volume due to collapse	
Pleural effusion	Lung cancer, lymphoma, metastases from cancers of breast and gut and other solid tumors	
Pericardial effusion	Tumor invades or irritates the surface of the pericardium and may lead to cardiac tamponade Lung cancer, breast cancer and lymphoma are the most common cancers causing pericardial effusion	Increase in heart rate Pulse is low in volume and fast Pulsus paradoxus
Lymphangitis carcinomatosa	Diffuse infiltration of lymphatic vessels by malignant disease Lung cancer, but may also originate from metastatic cancers, particularly of breast, gut and prostate.	Pulmonary congestion Difficult diagnosis to make and frequently underrecognized

Evaluation of multiple symptoms is done by the Edmonton Symptom Assessment System (ESAS) for nine cancer-related symptoms (see Appendix 1); the Support Team Assessment Schedule (STAS), with a five- or seven-point scale, measures dyspnea in terms of intensity, frequency and interference with activity.

Dyspnea alone can be evaluated by a visual analog scale (VAS), verbal rating scale or Likert-type scale. Recently, the Cancer Dyspnea Scale (CDS) has been validated in lung cancer patients for measuring dyspnea.

Treatment

Where appropriate, treatment of any underlying cause, such as anemia, infection or pulmonary embolism, should be given, and some patients may benefit from a specific anticancer treatment. There is evidence that patients with no apparent lung disease can suffer breathlessness, probably as a result of respiratory muscle weakness due to severe cachexia. Therefore, the majority of patients require symptomatic treatment based on the clinical characteristics of their breathlessness.

Accurate diagnosis of the causes of the dyspnea is required for etiological treatment, and multiple causes of dyspnea are often present and should generally be treated simultaneously.

Treatments of underlying physical causes of malignant dyspnea are given in Tables 11.2 and 11.3.

The pharmacological treatments for dyspnea are oxygen, bronchodilators, corticosteroids, antibiotics and opioids. One retrospective study at a medical center specializing in cancer assessed the resources used in the management of dyspnea due to lung cancer in 45 patients. The most common therapies administered in the emergency department were oxygen (31%), β_2 agonists (19%), antibiotics (12%) and opioids (11%).

Oxygen

Supplemental oxygen is the most commonly prescribed therapy to relieve dyspnea, but only a limited number of studies have shown a beneficial effect of oxygen therapy. Oxygen has been shown to be effective in reducing dyspnea in patients who are hypoxic and dyspneic at rest. The therapeutic value of oxygen therapy in other groups of patients with dyspnea is unclear. It is uncertain whether oxygen is better than air for relieving dyspnea in patients with advanced cancer. A prospective, double-blind, crossover trial studied the effects of supplemental oxygen on the intensity of dyspnea in 14 patients

Table 11.2 *Physical causes of dyspnea and their treatment*

Diagnosis	Possible treatments of underlying cause	Urgent management required?
Upper airway obstruction	Corticosteroids* Debulking of intraluminal lesions by endobronchial therapies Stenting of extrinsic compression Radiotherapy	Yes – if diagnosis suspected, give intravenous corticosteroids and emergency admission to hospital
Acute superior vena cava obstruction	Corticosteroids* Radiotherapy Chemotherapy for sensitive tumors Stenting of superior vena cava Thrombolysis	Yes – if diagnosis suspected, give intravenous corticosteroids and emergency admission to hospital
Pericardial effusion	Aspiration	If evidence of tamponade
Pleural effusion	Aspiration*; if recurrent consider pleurodesis	Possibly
Bronchial obstruction causing lung collapse	Corticosteroids* Radiotherapy Chemotherapy Endobronchial therapies	Possibly
Lymphangitis carcinomatosa	Corticosteroids* Chemotherapy for sensitive tumors	No

* Possible primary care treatments.

Table 11.3 Recommendations for palliation of cough and dyspnea

	Level of evidence	Grade of recommendation
Correctable causes of dyspnea (pleural effusion, coexisting COPD, airway obstruction)	Poor	C
Pharmacological treatment (oxygen, bronchodilators, corticosteroids, antibiotics, opioids)	Poor	C
Nonpharmacological treatment (patient education, breathing control, activity pacing, relaxation techniques)	Poor	C
For patients who continue to have cough, opioids are the best cough suppressants and should be used	Fair	C
Thoracentesis for drainage in patients with pleural effusion	Fair	C
Repeated thoracentesis for recurrent malignant pleural effusions in patients with NSCLC, poor PS and limited life expectancy	Fair	C
Pleurodesis after thoracentesis for recurring malignant pleural effusions in patients with NSCLC and better PS	Good	B
Systemic chemotherapy for malignant pleural effusions in patients with SCLC	Good	B
Bronchoscopy is needed in patients with central airway obstruction (to determine the type of airway obstruction)	Fair	B
Endobronchial therapy in patients with central airway obstruction (laser, electrocautorization, APC and/or insertion of stent)	Poor	C

APC, argon plasma coagulation; COPD, chronic obstructive pulmonary disease; NSCLC, non-small cell lung cancer; PS, performance status; SCLC: small cell lung cancer.

Grade of recommendation: (A) there is evidence of type I or consistent findings from multiple studies of types II, III or IV; (B) there is evidence of types II, III or IV and findings are generally consistent; (C) there is evidence of types II, III, or IV but findings are inconsistent; (D) there is little or no systematic empirical evidence.

with advanced cancer. The results showed that 12 patients consistently preferred oxygen to air, and patients reported little or no benefit from air compared with moderate to much benefit from oxygen. Irrespective of the oxygenation status, supplemental oxygen therapy should be considered if patients with lung cancer have dyspnea.

Bronchodilators

Patients with a history of reversible airway disease, chronic obstructive pulmonary disease (COPD) or symptoms of wheeze may benefit from bronchodilators. A prospective study of 100 terminally ill cancer patients (49 with lung cancer) showed that the potentially correctable causes of dyspnea included bronchospasm (in 52%) and hypoxia (in 40%). It is important to ensure that bronchodilator therapy is optimized if the patient has obstructive airways disease.

Corticosteroids

The role of systemic corticosteroids relieving dyspnea due to lung cancer is limited, but they are commonly used even if there are no controlled studies to support their use. As is the case with bronchodilator therapy, patients with obstructive lung disease may benefit from treatment with systemic corticosteroids by decreased mucus production and inflammatory changes in the airway mucosa. In one study, 50% of patients had a factor of bronchospasm contributing to their dyspnea. All patients may be given a trial of an oral corticosteroid, either for an anti-inflammatory effect or to reduce peritumoral edema, unless there is a contraindication. Because dexamethasone is used empirically for dyspnea, it is important to taper to the minimum effective dose that controls symptoms. There is little evidence to guide the best starting dose of oral dexamethasone, but a dose of 8–12 mg/day is commonly used.

Opioids

If tachypnea is also a central feature of respiratory difficulties, opioids are useful to decrease central respiratory drive. Smaller doses and dose increments of opioids than those used for pain relief are given and titrated to subjective response. It is not clear whether all opioids are equally effective in decreasing dyspnea perception in patients with lung cancer. In a study of 104 patients with lung cancer, opioids administered to treat pain did not decrease dyspnea. The relation between opioids and respiration is not simple; if used inappropriately, opioids can induce respiratory depression, which is determined by pathophysiology, prior exposure to opioids, rate and route of dose titration, and coexisting pathology. However, low-dose oral opioids can improve breathlessness, sometimes dramatically, although the precise mechanism of action is unknown. The dose of opioid can be titrated in the same way as when used for pain control, but at lower doses and smaller increments. In patients without prior exposure to opioids, 2.5 mg oral morphine every 4 hours may be sufficient. A dose of 5–10 mg every 4 hours or as required should be used for patients who have previously been taking a weak opioid, e.g. codeine. In patients on regular morphine, the dose may be increased by 30–50% every 2–3 days until symptoms are controlled or adverse effects prevent further dose escalation.

Benzodiazepines

These drugs are effective in low doses, particularly in patients whose anxiety augments dyspnea, although benefit in patients with no apparent anxiety is also observed, probably because of sedation and muscle relaxation. Lorazepam 0.5–2 mg given sublingually can be useful in acute dyspnea. If continued treatment is required, diazepam 5 mg daily is started, and the dose slowly titrated to obtain the maximum response with minimum sedation.

Physiotherapy

Breathlessness often is an emotion-loaded experience associated with fear, anxiety, helplessness, panic or depression. Optimal control of dyspnea is achieved when drug treatment is given in conjunction with physiotherapy, counseling and the provision of practical aids for daily living. Patients may have feelings of impending death during the acute dyspneic attack. They should be advised of measures that they may initiate to allow them to regain control: stop (try to stay calm), purse lips, drop (relax shoulders, back, neck and arms) and flop (concentrate on breathing out slowly). A multicenter randomized controlled trial was conducted in 119 patients with lung cancer or mesothelioma who had completed first-line treatment and reported dyspnea. Patients in the intervention group attended a weekly nursing clinic for up to 8 weeks. Various strategies were used: breathing control, activity pacing, relaxation techniques and psychosocial support, in addition to standard treatment for dyspnea. The group assigned to intervention by nurses improved significantly at 8 weeks in breathlessness, performance status, physical and emotional status compared with the control group. Controlled breathing techniques included positioning, pursed-lip breathing (PLB), breathing exercises and coordinated breathing training. Pacing of breathing with activity, energy-conservation techniques and home modification can maintain the patient's basic activities of daily living.

Cough

Prevalence

Cough is a normal but complex physiological mechanism that protects the airways and lungs by removing mucus and foreign matter from the larynx, trachea and bronchi; it is under both voluntary and involuntary control. Pathological cough is common in malignant and nonmalignant disease. Breathlessness can trigger cough and vice versa. Persistent cough can also precipitate vomiting, exhaustion, chest or abdominal pain, rib fracture, syncope and insomnia. Cough has a prevalence of 47–86% in lung cancer and 23–37% in general cancer patients. Cough of moderate to severe intensity occurred in 13% of general cancer patients and in 17–48% of lung cancer patients. Few studies have quantitatively examined the distress caused by cough in cancer patients. In one series of 240 cancer patients, of whom 21.3% had lung cancer, cough was present in 33%. Among all patients, 13% had moderate to severe cough, and 18% of all patients suffered from severe distress due to cough. In lung cancer, cough is a frequent and distressing symptom that can be dry or produce sputum. Among the initial symptoms of lung cancer, cough is present in more than 65% and productive cough in more than 25% of patients.

Cough can be classified as productive cough in a patient able to cough effectively, productive cough in a patient not able to cough effectively, and nonproductive cough.

Etiology

Chronic cough is due to multiple causes in the general population. In cancer, it is likely that multiple causes and hence multiple mechanisms are responsible. The causes of cough in cancer are shown in Table 11.4.

Treatment

In the general population, the treatment of cough is highly successful if the underlying cause is identified and treated. In cancer patients, the identification of a specific cause may be hampered by the burden of investigations, and treatment of cough can be categorized into specific treatment of the underlying causes, enhancing effectiveness of cough when indicated and suppression of cough. Specific treatments of cough are given in Table 11.5.

■ *Opioids.:* These are the best cough suppressants in patients with lung cancer, especially in advanced stages, when standard nonopioid cough

Table 11.4 *Causes of cough*

Non-malignant	Cancer-related
Postnasal drip syndrome (PNDS)	Major airway or endobronchial lesions
Asthma	Pleural disease: effusion, mesothelioma
Gastroesophageal reflux disease (GERD)	Lung parenchymal infiltration
Chronic bronchitis	Aspiration (e.g. head and neck tumors,
Postinfectious	tracheoesophageal fistula, vocal
Angiotensin-converting enzyme	cord paralysis)
(ACE) inhibitors	Lymphangitis carcinomatosis
Eosinophilic bronchitis	Pericardial effusion
Bronchiectasis	Radiation-induced fibrosis
Heart failure	Chemotherapy-induced fibrosis
	Postobstructive pneumonia
	Microembolism

Table 11.5 *Specific causes and treatments of cough*

Cause	Treatment
Endobronchial tumors	Corticosteroids, laser, cryotherapy
Tracheoesophageal fistula	Stent
Lymphangitis carcinomatosis	Corticosteroids
Post-irradiation lung damage	Corticosteroids
Pleural and pericardial effusion	Fluid aspiration
Aspiration pneumonia	Antibiotics, prevention of aspiration
Congestive heart failure	Diuretics
Asthma	Bronchodilators, corticosteroids
Postnasal drip syndrome (PNDS)	Antihistamines
Gastroesophageal reflux (GERD)	H_2 blocker, proton pump inhibitor, diet modification
Eosinophilic bronchitis	Corticosteroids

suppressants are not effective. Codeine is the most widely used opioid. A double-blind randomized controlled trial compared the therapeutic efficacy and the tolerability of a 7-day treatment with levodropropizine drops (75 mg three times a day) and dihydrocodeine drops (10 mg three times a day) on nonproductive cough in 140 adults with primary lung cancer or lung metastases. Efficacy was assessed by cough severity scores, the number of night awakenings due to cough, and overall estimate of antitussive efficacy. Subjective cough severity was significantly reduced during treatment with levodropropizine and dihydrocodeine, and the antitussive effect and its time profile were similar for both drugs. Moreover, according to the investigators' evaluation, both levodropropizine and dihydrocodeine treatment produced a significant decrease in cough severity. Concurrently with the relief of cough, the number of night awakenings was decreased by both drugs. However, the percentage of patients experiencing somnolence in the group receiving levodropropizine (8%) was significantly lower than in the dihydrocodeine group (22%). These results confirm the antitussive effectiveness of levodropropizine and suggest a more favorable benefit/risk profile than for dihydrocodeine. It should be noted that levodropropizine is not available in the USA.

■ *Nonopioid cough suppressants.* These may be active in a small group of patients with advanced lung cancer. Occasionally, opioid-resistant cough may respond to agents such as the peripherally acting nonopioid drug benzonatate.

■ *Bronchodilators.* Bronchospasm can cause or contribute to cough. In patients with lung cancer and underlying bronchospastic obstructive airways disease, standard bronchodilator therapy may help to alleviate cough. One study tested the role of inhaled sodium cromoglycate in 20 patients with NSCLC and cough resistant to conventional treatment. In a double-blind trial, patients were randomized to receive either inhaled sodium cromoglycate or placebo. The results showed that inhaled sodium cromoglycate reduced cough in all patients with NSCLC.

■ *Corticosteroids.* There are no studies of the effect of corticosteroids on cough in lung cancer patients. If cough is induced by radiation, high-dose corticosteroid therapy may be used.

■ *Inhaled lidocaine.* There are no studies of the effect of inhaled lidocaine on cough in patients with lung cancer.

■ *Bronchoscopic methods to palliate dyspnea and cough.* Most patients with dyspnea caused by central airway obstruction also complain of cough. The severity of dyspnea is dependent on the extent of luminal involvement of the airway, and the presence or absence of underlying conditions such as COPD, cardiac failure, or loss of lung tissue due to previous lung surgery. Extraluminal tumor compression of the major airways, intraluminal tumor growth or a combination of both can cause central airway obstruction. Perhaps the most important aspect of the management of these patients is to determine the anatomical type of airway involvement by bronchoscopy. Bronchoscopy will also determine the feasibility of endoscopic therapy. The degree of dyspnea and respiratory distress should dictate the appropriate endobronchial therapy: debulking of intraluminal tumor (usually with rigid bronchoscopy), balloon dilation, laser therapy, electrocautery, cryotherapy, argon plasma coagulation (APC), endobronchial irradiation, or intraluminal stent placement. All of these therapeutic techniques provide significant relief of dyspnea and cough in the majority of patients.

Acute respiratory failure

Prevalence

Two important pathological entities may be responsible for acute respiratory failure: adult respiratory distress syndrome (ARDS) and airways obstruction. About 19% of cancer patients die of respiratory failure. Up to 76% of all cancer patients who require mechanical ventilation have a fatal outcome. Acute respiratory failure occurring in bone-marrow transplant patients carries a mortality rate of 59–81%.

Adult respiratory distress syndrome (ARDS)

ARDS is the most common reason for admission to the intensive care unit (ICU) from an oncology service.

Etiology

ARDS has multiple etiologies:

- infection is the most frequent respiratory complication determining acute pulmonary insufficiency
- aggressive multimodality therapy with acute lung injury and drug toxicity
- aspiration pneumonia, tumor emboli, massive tissue necrosis, diffuse intravascular clotting, massive transfusion, drug and radiation toxicity, and opportunistic infections
- all-*trans*-retinoic acid (ATRA) therapy in patients with promyelocytic leukemia (retinoic acid syndrome)
- gemcitabine therapy in the perioperative period in patients undergoing lung resection.

Diagnosis

This is on the basis of:
- determination of the cause of ARDS
- progressive hypoxemia

- radiographic evidence of pulmonary congestion and/or multilobar infiltrates
- non-cardiogenic pulmonary edema
- reduced lung compliance and progressive intrapulmonary shunting.

All criteria do not have to be present simultaneously for diagnosis of ARDS.

Clinical features

- Dyspnea and rapid shallow respiration are present.
- Cough (usually nonproductive) is absent or feeble due to generalized weakness; sputum may be evident in acute bacterial pneumonia.
- Cyanosis, intercostal muscle retractions and accessory respiratory muscle use may be present. The patient may be agitated, confused or obtunded.
- Endobronchial aspiration may produce copious amounts of serosanguineous fluid, but frankly bloody fluid should suggest other causes.
- Initially, chest examination is often normal, but as ARDS progresses, rales and ronchi may be heard. It is not uncommon for patients to develop pleural effusions after intubation because of ventilator effects on thoracic hemodynamics. In ARDS, extensive multilobar pulmonary infiltrates develop over 12–24 hours.
- Arterial blood gas analysis will show a progressive and severe decline in oxygen saturation (SaO_2) and partial pressure in arterial blood (PaO_2).

Treatment

Treatment is primarily supportive and should be directed at the underlying cause (Table 11.6).

- Restoration of oxygen saturation (SaO_2 at 95% and PaO_2 at 60 mmHg) usually by intubation and ventilator assistance. In ARDS, high inspired oxygen concentrations (FiO_2 up to 1.0) are often required to maintain adequate SaO_2/PaO_2 levels, because of the loss of alveolar compliance and extensive right-to-left shunting. The use of positive end-expiratory pressure (PEEP) ventilation has been shown to be effective in reversing arterial hypoxemia.
- Maintainance of blood pressure and tissue perfusion by administration of intravenous fluids (especially in septic shock). Overhydration may result in worsening of respiratory failure.
- Vasopressors are required if hypotension does not respond to a fluid challenge.
- Diuretics and digoxin are usually ineffective, since pulmonary edema of ARDS is noncardiogenic.

Table 11.6 *Treatment of acquired respiratory distress syndrome*

Oxygen	S_aO_2 95% and P_aO_2 60 mmHg
Hypotension tendency	Intravenous fluids
Hypotension does not respond to a fluid challenge	Vasopressors
Sepsis suspected	Appropriate antibiotics
Disseminated intravascular coagulation (DIC)	Heparin and factor replacement

- The use of a Swan–Ganz catheter is critical, particularly in patients with underlying cardiovascular disease and those requiring high levels of positive-pressure ventilation or large volumes of fluid.
- Appropriate antibiotics should be administered if sepsis is suspected.
- Diffuse intravascular clotting should be treated with heparin and factor replacement therapy.

Airways obstruction

Incidence

It is estimated that malignant airway obstruction affects up to 80 000 people annually in the USA. Central airway obstructions located at the hypopharynx, larynx and trachea to carina are defined as upper airway obstructions, and those at the main stem and lobar bronchi and their more distal radicals as lower airway obstructions. Clinical differentiation between upper and lower airway obstructions can be difficult. Obstructive lesions can cause cough, dyspnea, wheezing, infection, atelectasis, respiratory failure and death.

Clinical presentation

- prolonged inspiratory phase with stridor and retraction of the intercostal muscles in 85% of patients (tracheal syndrome)
- anxiety, diaphoresis and tachycardia
- progression of asphyxiation resulting in cyanosis and decreased consciousness with development of bradycardia and disappearance of stridor.

Evaluation and treatment

Upper airway obstruction

Etiology

- multiple benign causes, including aspiration of food or other foreign bodies, tracheal stenosis, tracheomalacia and edema
- tumors involving the base of the tongue, hypopharynx, larynx, thyroid or mediastinum and primary carcinoma of the trachea, adenomas and sarcomas.

Evaluation

- A rapid evaluation must be performed:
  - Ensure that no foreign body was inhaled.
  - In cancer patients, the most likely cause is the tumor mass or edema.
- Arterial blood gases are not useful in the evaluation of upper airway obstruction.
- Spirometry and chest radiography are relatively insensitive and time-consuming.
- Emergency visualization of the larynx by an otolaryngologist or anesthesiologist is indicated in order to pass an endotracheal tube.

Treatment

- The decision to intervene is based solely on the clinical condition of the patient.
- An emergency low tracheotomy with placement of a long tracheostomy tube should be performed (this technique is effective for lesions involving the hypopharynx, larynx and upper third of the trachea).
- Adjunctive therapy includes intravenous corticosteroids to reduce edema, humidified oxygen and bronchodilators.
- Definitive treatment depends on the underlying condition:
  - Chemotherapy-sensitive neoplasms (lymphoma, germ cell tumors, or small cell lung cancer) will be treated with chemotherapy.
  - Other cancers will be treated by radiotherapy, endoscopic laser, siliconized tracheal stents, or surgical resection for some obstructing low tracheal lesions.

Lower airway obstruction

Etiology

■ primary carcinoma of the lung (the most frequent cause)
■ endobronchial metastases
■ AIDS-related Kaposi's sarcoma.

The symptoms are cough, hemoptysis, wheezing, fever, dyspnea and obstructive pneumonitis.

Evaluation

■ radiographic studies (including expiratory films)
■ bronchoscopy with cytology, and biopsy.

Treatment

■ Surgical, radiotherapeutic or chemotherapeutic management, depending on the patient and tumor type, is employed.
■ For recurrent endobronchial obstruction, laser endoscopy and endobronchial brachytherapy as complementary techniques may be beneficial.

Hemoptysis

Hemoptysis is defined as coughing up of blood. The most common causes are chronic bronchitis, cancer and tuberculosis.

Prevalence

Hemoptysis occurs in 20% of patients with lung cancer, and approximately 3% of patients with lung cancer develop massive terminal hemoptysis. In 18% of patients, massive hemoptysis was associated with squamous cell carcinoma. In recent decades, the frequency of bleeding caused by cancer has increased while that caused by tuberculosis has decreased.

The main source of bleeding is superficial mucosal inflammation or erosion of the bronchial arterial system. Massive hemoptysis (MH) is defined as expectoration of at least 100–600 ml of blood in 24 hours. Blood clots may cause respiratory insufficiency by obstruction of airways. The prognosis of MH is very poor; the mortality rate is 59% in patients with lung cancer.

The causes of hemoptysis in cancer patients are shown in Table 11.7.

Table 11.7 *Causes of hemoptysis in cancer patients*

Lung cancer	Communication between tumor and vessels
Tumor involving major airway	Tracheal tumor, pulmonary carcinoid, endobronchial metastases
Paramalignant causes	Cancer-related coagulopathy, thrombo-cytopenia, disseminated intravascular coagulopathy, pulmonary embolism
Nonmalignant causes	Infection, tuberculosis, bronchiectasis, fungal pneumonia in hematological malignancies

Diagnostic and differential diagnosis

Evaluation is by medical history, physical examination and specific investigation of underlying disease (radiography, bronchoscopy or laboratory tests).

Differential diagnoses are as follows:

■ bleeding from the upper airway (sinusitis, nasal polyps, and laryngeal and nasopharyngeal neoplasms)
■ bleeding due to aspiration from the gastrointestinal tract (nausea and vomiting).
■ pseudohemoptysis due to pigmentation by microbes such as *Serratia marcescens* or medication (e.g. oxidized isoetharine).

Management

■ Surgical resection of the bleeding lobe is done when hemoptysis is a symptom at the time of lung cancer diagnosis in patients amenable to surgery with curative intent.
■ Endotracheal intubation is done with a single lumen tube in patients with MH. Bronchoscopy is useful to identify the source of bleeding. Endobroncheal treatment consists of continuous suction to collapse the segment. This management is used when there is one location of bleeding but no direct source. Epinephrine solution $1/10\,000$ is instilled in the segment.
■ Balloons may be used to control the bleeding by tamponade.
■ ANd–YAG laser can be used for photocoagulation.
■ Electrocautery has the same efficiency (60%) as the laser.
■ For endobronchial cancer visualized by bronchoscopy, bronchial artery embolization is beneficial.
■ For unresectable lung cancer, external-beam radiotherapy can be applied.

- Pharmacological approach:
    - tranexamic acid 1000–1500 mg × 3/day
    - prednisone 40–60 mg × 1/day or dexamethasone 6–9 mg × 1/day with dose tapering according to response.

Death rales

Death rales (death rattle) occur in the terminal stage of diseases such as cancer or other progressive incurable disorders. If death rales occur, death may be imminent. In the final hours, most patients are semiconscious or unconscious, unable to swallow saliva, and unable to cough up mucus from the trachea. Breathing with partial obstruction caused by these secretions in the central airways or glottic area causes a noisy respiration called the 'death rattle'. Other symptoms of this terminal syndrome are lack of communication, cough, increased or irregular respiratory rate and sometimes Cheyne–Stokes respiration; the pulse becomes weaker or not palpable and the body temperature may initially increase due to vasodilation.

Prevention of death rales is by an anticholinergic drug (e.g. hyoscine) administered as a single parenteral dose or by continuous infusion, reposition of the patient or suction with a soft catheter. The family should be informed that the patient is not suffering and offered psychological support.

Further reading

Davis LC: Clinical review, ABC of palliative care: breathlessness, cough and other respiratory problems. BMJ 1997; 315: 931–4.

Doyle D, Hanks G, Cherny NI, Calman K: Oxford Textbook of Palliative Medicine, 3rd edn. Oxford: Oxford University Press, 2004.

Dudgeon DJ, Lertzman M: Dyspnoea in the advanced cancer patient. J Pain Symptom Manage 1998; 16: 212–9.

Kvale PA, Simoff M, Prakash UBS: Palliative care. Chest; 2003; 123: 284S–311S.

PRODIGY Guidance: Palliative care 2005. Dyspnoea. www.prodigy.nhs.uk.

Vonk-Noordegraaf A, Postmus PE, Sutedja TG: Central airways obstruction. Chest 2001; 120: 1811–14

Yeung S-C J, Escalante CP: Acute suffocation by malignant airway obstruction. Cancer Medicine Section 42, Oncologic Emergencies. Hamilton, Canada: BC Decker, 2000: 158.

Genitourinary problems in advanced cancer

12

M Laufer, U Lindner
Chaim Sheba Medical Center, Israel

Urinary obstruction
Prevalence

There are no estimations of the prevalence of urinary tract obstruction secondary to advanced malignancy. However, obstruction of the upper urinary tract, primarily the ureters, is common in a variety of cancers. Sometimes obstruction is bilateral, and patients may present with simultaneous or sequential obstruction resulting in anuria and renal failure.

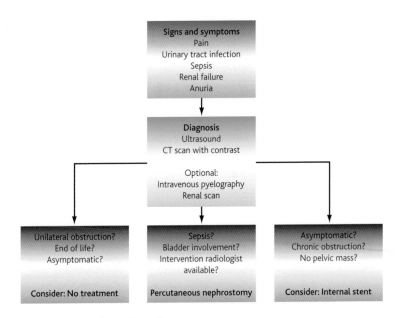

Figure 12.1 Approach to urinary obstruction

Etiology

Malignancies that may cause ureteral obstruction include urological, gynecological and colorectal cancers, lymphomas, sarcomas, and germ-cell tumors, as well as metastases from breast, lung and other cancers. Obstruction may be due to tumor compression, retroperitoneal adenopathies or direct tumor invasion. It is strongly recommended that patients with pelvic and retroperitoneal cancers be closely monitored for evidence of acute or chronic ureteral obstruction. Early recognition of obstruction and tailored intervention can improve the patient's quality of life and prevent life-threatening complications.

Clinical manifestations

Urinary obstruction may present with acute 'renal colic-like' signs and symptoms (Figure 12.1). These include flank pain and tenderness, nausea, vomiting, fever, chills, hematuria and oliguria/anuria (in patients with single-kidney or bilateral obstruction). More frequently, due to the slow growth of

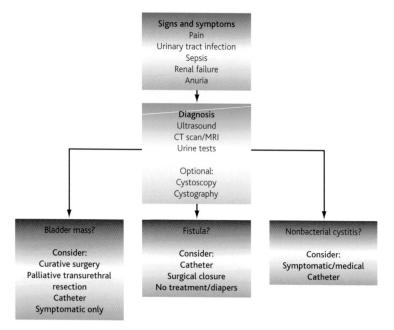

Figure 12.2 Approach to urinary symptoms

tumor mass, ureteral obstruction is mostly asymptomatic with only mild flank tenderness. Laboratory tests may show rising blood urea nitrogen (BUN) and creatinine compared with baseline levels.

Diagnostic procedures

Diagnosis is based primarily on imaging studies. These include ultrasound of the urinary system with hydronephrosis and hydroureter, and computed tomography (CT) scan, which can demonstrate more accurately the etiology and level of obstruction. With both modalities, it is very important to estimate the thickness of the renal parenchyma and to compare the results with previous scans. In equivocal cases, a formal intravenous pyelography (IVP) and/or renal scan may be necessary. When renal function allows, CT urography is the modality of choice.

Treatment

In the majority of patients, due to the extent of disease and/or metastatic spread, surgical approach is a viable option. However, the surgical treatment should be considered on an individual basis in some patients during remission, mainly in colon and cervical cancers. Palliative radiotherapy is only rarely successful in relieving external ureteral obstruction. Obstruction caused by germ-cell tumors, lymphomas, and bladder and prostate cancers, is frequently resolved by adequate chemotherapy or hormonal therapy.

Symptomatic urinary obstruction accompanied by urinary tract infection, sepsis, pain or acute renal failure usually requires emergency drainage (Figure 12.2). Options include percutaneous nephrostomy (usually by an interventional radiologist) or retrograde stenting of the ureter (endoscopic urological procedure). Drainage should be tailored to the individual patient according to multiple factors, including gender, level of obstruction, presence of sepsis and urinary bladder involvement. In general, in hospitals where an experienced interventional radiologist is available, percutaneous nephrostomy is the method of choice in the patient with advanced cancer, offering a higher success rate, better tolerance by the patient and easier exchange procedure.

Some cancer patients present with asymptomatic hydronephrosis on routine scans or a slowly rising creatinine level. These patients can be treated with retrograde ureteral stenting. However, in these cases, a 'no-touch technique' should also be considered, and the pros and cons of nephrostomy or internal stenting should be discussed with the patient and family in relation to prognosis and quality of life. In many patients with unilateral obstruction, drainage of an obstructed kidney is not necessary.

Exchange of internal ureteral stents is necessary every 3–6 months. In most patients, several days after insertion of a percutaneous nephrostomy, replacement of the nephrostomy with an internal ureteral stent should be attempted to obviate the need for an external urinary bag.

Radiation-induced hemorrhagic cystitis
Prevalence

Radiation-induced hemorrhagic cystitis (HC) symptoms may vary from mild intermittent nuisance to a true medical emergency. The precise prevalence is not known, but it seems to be declining due to better radiation techniques.

Etiology

Radiation to the pelvis for curative or palliative intent may cause radiation cystitis and sometimes gross hematuria. Radiation for cervical, rectal and prostate cancers is the most common cause. Radiation for bladder cancer as part of bladder preservation protocols may also result in HC, which should be suspected in any cancer patient ever treated by radiotherapy to the bladder region. Other causes of hematuria (e.g. stones and ureter or kidney masses) in the upper urinary tract should be ruled out. Another cause of hematuria, especially in women, is bacterial cystitis.

Diagnosis

Definite diagnosis is made after ruling out other causes and demonstration of typical mucosal bleedings and edema by cystoscopy.

Treatment

The initial treatment in patients with acute symptoms due to blood clots in the bladder consists of evacuation of clots and drainage with a three-way irrigation catheter. This simple procedure with continuous irrigation for a few days often resolves the episode of bleeding without further treatment. If bleeding does not stop with this procedure, the urologist can sometimes fulgurate bleeding points in the bladder by a cystoscope.

More resistant and recurrent episodes may be palliated by bladder irrigation with estrogens and other clotting-enhancing agents and formaldehyde. Surgical or radiological interventions are sometimes needed. In recent years, hyperbaric oxygen has shown encouraging results in several small series.

Frequency–urgency–urinary incontinence–dysuria

Prevalence

Frequency, urgency, urinary incontinence and dysuria are all related symptoms that reflect a spectrum of bladder morbidity. The prevalence of those symptoms is very high, especially in patients with primary pelvic malignancies or metastases to the pelvis.

Etiology

In many patients, bladder symptoms may be unrelated to the underlying cancer. Diagnoses such as benign prostatic hyperplasia (BPH) and reactive bladder or stress incontinence are common in elderly men and women respectively.

When related to advanced cancer, bladder symptoms may be the result of cancer therapy, such as surgery with injury to the bladder, radiation or chemotherapy. Other causes may be extension of tumor into the bladder, pressure outside the bladder by a tumor mass, and vesicovaginal or vesicorectal fistulae. It is also important to rule out paradoxical incontinence (overflow bladder) as a result of chronic urinary retention.

Diagnostic procedures

Basic evaluation includes urinalysis, urine culture, renal function tests and ultrasound of the lower urinary tract, including determination of residual urine volume. Routine staging imaging such as CT scan or magnetic resonance imaging (MRI) of the pelvis may reveal tumor mass at or inside the bladder. Cystoscopy is necessary when a mass in the bladder is suspected from imaging. Diagnosis of fistulae is based on combination of cystoscopy, cystography and other individualized tests.

Treatment

Treatment of a tumor mass outside or inside the bladder depends on the patient's primary cancer and prognosis. In some patients with colorectal cancer, surgery is warranted for solitary recurrence or metastases. When prognosis is good, one may consider surgical urinary diversion as part of pelvic exenteration.

In patients with advanced cancer in whom curative treatment is not possible, palliative transurethral resection of the bladder mass can alleviate bleeding and other debilitating symptoms. In these patients, a permanent urethral or suprapubic catheter can solve severe bladder symptoms.

Fistulae are treated according to the patient's prognosis. In some patients, a long-term, indwelling catheter may cause spontaneous closure of the fistula.

In radiation- or chemotherapy-induced cystitis, symptomatic therapy with antimuscarinic or tricyclic agents may relieve symptoms.

BPH and chronic urinary retention should be treated as in noncancer patients.

Neurological problems in advanced cancer

13

N Chamseddine, M Tohfé
Division of Haematology–Oncology, Saint George Hospital,
University Medical Center, Lebanon

Introduction

Disorders of the central or peripheral nervous system affect approximately 15% of patients with cancer. The disorders usually appear in patients with advanced metastatic disease, although they may be the first symptom of cancer. Regardless of whether neurological complications occur early or late in the course of the disease, they threaten the quality of the patient's life by causing such distressing symptoms as dementia, paralysis and pain; in addition, neurological dysfunction itself shortens survival.

Neurological diseases can be direct effects of the tumor, infection, metabolic abnormalities or toxicity of therapy, or of the paraneoplastic syndromes frequently seen with certain tumors, such as small-cell lung cancer. In this chapter, we review certain neurological problems related to cancer.

Raised intracranial pressure
Etiology

Intracranial pressure depends on systemic blood pressure, venous pressure and intrathoracic pressure; its range is 5–15 mmHg. In patients with intracranial space-occupying lesions (brain tumors, metastases, edema), the pressure may rise to 15–22 mmHg without significant impact on the neurological condition of the patient. When it reaches 30 mmHg, brain activity decreases and signs of hypoperfusion occur; when it reaches 60 mmHg, death occurs.

Raised intracranial pressure can cause herniation of the brain with displacement within the skull. Central herniation causes compression of the diencephalon and brainstem; uncal herniation is displacement of the temporal lobe or that part of it under the cerebellar tentorium, and cerebellar herniation displaces cerebellar structures through the occipital foramen.

Symptoms

Clinical findings depend on the velocity of the rise in intracranial pressure. Symptoms and signs are given in Table 13.1.

Diagnosis

■ Clinical neurological examination may show neurological deficits in cranial nerves. Papillary eye edema may be present in raised intracranial pressure.

■ Electroencephalography (EEG) may show typical waves due to a sudden rise in intracranial pressure.

■ Computed tomography (CT) scan of the brain may show intracranial lesions and edema.

■ Magnetic resonance imaging (MRI) of the brain may show intracranial lesions and edema.

Treatment

Raised intracranial pressure is a potentially lethal condition. Conservative treatment aims to maintain cerebral perfusion and reduce vasogenic edema.

■ Position of patient: head should be at least 30° above the heart.

■ Hyperventilation: reduction of P_{CO2} and vasoconstriction decrease intracranial blood flow.

■ Control of arterial blood pressure.

■ Hypertonic infusions: intravenous mannitol (mannitol 20%, 1 g/kg in 15–30 minutes every 12 hours for 3 days) decreases intracranial pressure and edema

■ Corticosteroids: dexamethasone: 4 mg × 4/day or 96 mg/day.

Prognosis

Prognosis is poor if the cause of the raised intracranial pressure cannot be treated by surgery (primary brain tumors and metastases), radiotherapy (brain metastases) or systemic treatment (chemosensitive tumors or metastases).

Seizures

Introduction

Epilepsy refers to recurrent seizures that reflect the aberrant electrical activity of cerebral cortical neurons. Convulsion refers to a seizure in which motor manifestations predominate. Seizures in a patient with cancer can be caused by the tumor itself, by metabolic disturbances, by radiation injury, by

Table 13.1 *Symptoms and signs of raised intracranial pressure*

General
Altered state of consciousness, agitation, delirium
Headache, neck pain
Focal or generalized seizures
Cerebral fits (opistotonus)
Decerebration (hypertonus, extensions and intrarotation of limbs)
Coma, death
Amaurosis fugax, midriasis
Cranial nerve paralysis (II, IV, VI), conjugated eye deviation
Nystagmus, dysphagia
Myoclonus of face and limb muscles
Dysarthria, dysphagia
Pyramidal signs, paresthesia
Cardiovascular or respiratory disturbances, yawning
Hypertermia, face cyanosis, flushing, pallor, sweating
Nausea, vomiting, hiccup, sialorrhea, diarrhea, incontinence
Central herniation
Decreased level of consciousness
Cheyne–Stokes respiration
Myosis, presence or absence of doll's-eye phenomenon
Paratonic rigidity
Coma, ataxic breathing
Uncal herniation
Initial homolateral midriasis; visual field defects
Decreased level of consciousness
Hyperventilation followed by Cheyne–Stokes respiration
Cerebral herniation
Occipital and frontal headache
Vomiting
Hiccup
Decreased consciousness
Cerebellar fits

cerebral infarctions, by chemotherapy-related encephalopathies or by central nervous system (CNS) infections. Metastatic disease in the CNS is the most common cause of seizures in patients with cancer. Seizures are a presenting symptom of CNS metastasis in 6–29% of patients. Approximately 10% of patients with CNS metastasis eventually develop seizures.

Classification

Seizures are classified by their EEG features as follows:

- Partial (focal) seizures, in which a specific focus can be identified.
  - Simple partial seizure: consciousness *is not* impaired. Patients may experience déjà vu and sensory, motor or autonomic symptoms. With motor involvement, patients are likely to exhibit hemifacial or hemibody twitching.
  - Complex partial seizure: consciousness *is* impaired. Patients may have automatic behaviors such as lip smacking, fumbling with clothes or even walking. Patients are amnestic for part of or the whole episode.
- Generalized seizures are bilateral and symmetric without focal onset.
  - Absence (petit mal): brief (2–10 seconds) lapse of consciousness without aura. Manifested by staring, eye blinking or lip smacking.
  - Clonic, tonic and tonic–clonic (grand mal): with or without aura, the patient abruptly loses consciousness and has a tonic, clonic or tonic–clonic convulsion, followed by postictal confusion.
  - Status epilepticus is a seizure (convulsive or otherwise) persisting more than 30 minutes or when a patient fails to return to normal consciousness between seizures. A seizure lasting more than 5 minutes puts a patient at increased risk of developing status epilepticus. Permanent brain damage starts in 30 minutes.

Etiology

Seizures result from electrical irritability of gray matter through many possible mechanisms, including CNS infection, congenital malformation, acquired metabolic disorder (hypoglycemia, uremia, hepatic encephalopathy, and disturbances of sodium, chloride, magnesium, calcium or pH), structural lesions (stroke, trauma, subarachnoid hemorrhage, subdural hematoma or tumors), gliosis from old brain injuries, new medications or medication withdrawal, drug or alcohol use or withdrawal, and familial epilepsy.

Rarely, cytotoxic drugs, such as methotrexate, vincristine, cisplatin, etoposide (high-dose), and busulfan (high-dose), can cause seizures.

Radionecrosis of the brain, the most common late delayed complication of radiotherapy, may cause seizures. There is a threshold near 6000 cGy above which radionecrosis becomes common.

Diagnosis

- History: ask questions to characterize accurately the start, middle and end of the seizure. Information from witnesses is essential. Ask about prior seizures, medications, fever, headache, circumstances precipitating events, history of drug abuse, ingestions and trauma.
- Physical examination: assess neurological (responsiveness, pupils, fundi, cranial nerves, and sensory, motor and reflex asymmetry), cardiovascular (blood pressure and perfusion) and pulmonary (cyanosis and irregular breathing) function. Check for breath odor (fruity indicates diabetic ketoacidosis or fetor hepaticus), rash, signs and symptoms of infection (sepsis and meningitis), signs of trauma, and cirrhosis.
- Laboratory tests: electrolytes, calcium, magnesium, glucose, blood urea level, blood cell count, liver function tests, anticonvulsant levels (if applicable), toxicology screen and sepsis workup, including lumbar puncture if indicated.
- EEG examination: this supports the diagnosis of seizures. Abnormal neuronal discharges are more frequent in the first few days after a seizure. Obtaining an EEG during this period improves sensitivity and the chances of electrically localizing a seizure focus. A normal EEG does not rule out a seizure disorder, and an abnormal EEG does not always mean epilepsy, because the EEG will generally be positive after a seizure but may revert to normal in 3–4 weeks.
- MRI: this is sensitive for structural brain lesions, including tumors, strokes and hippocampal sclerosis.

Differential diagnosis

- Syncope is global brain hypoperfusion secondary to decreased cardiac output or vasodilation.
- Pseudoseizures manifest psychological illness and are usually poorly stereotyped, varying in form and duration. Most epileptic seizures last less than 3 minutes, but pseudoseizures may have a much longer duration. They are much more likely to occur during times of stress and do not typically occur while alone or during dangerous activities.
- Transient ischemic attacks (TIA) are usually of relatively short duration. They are characterized by loss of neurological function and only rarely cause motor activity.

■ Migraine aura also causes a transient neurological dysfunction, but it does not manifest as motor activity. It can cause alterations in sensation, dexterity, balance, vision and alertness.

Prevention

There are no randomized trials showing that patients with brain metastases should receive prophylactic anticonvulsant treatment.

Treatment

If possible, an etiological treatment should be started:

■ In the case of cerebral edema producing mass effect, dexamethasone may give symptomatic relief.
■ Treatment of the underlying cause:
  – irradiation of metastatic lesions
  – correction of metabolic disturbances
  – discontinuation of the incriminated chemotherapeutic drug.

Symptomatic treatment is best as a single-drug therapy, because polypharmacy impairs drug effectiveness and increases side effects. Drugs of choice are carbamazepine, valproic acid and phenytoin for most simple-partial, complex-partial and generalized seizures, and valproic acid for absence seizures (Table 13.2). It is useful to control anticonvulsant levels after dose adjustment or when changing to/from some other drug with a known anti-convulsant interaction.

Status epilepticus

■ Manage airway: seizures may cause hypoxia, and treatment (benzodiazepines and phenobarbital) may cause apnea.
■ Correct the underlying metabolic problem if one is present.
■ Benzodiazepines:
  – lorazepam 0.1 mg/kg intravenously 2 mg/min up to 8 mg in adults

Table 13.2 Anticonvulsant treatment

Drug	Daily dose	Schedule	Plasma levels
Carbamazepine	400–1200 mg	q8–12 h	4–12 mg/ml
Phenytoin	4–8 mg/kg	q8–12 h	10–20 µg/ml
Valproic acid	1000–3000 mg	q12 h	50–100 mg/ml

- diazepam 0.1–0.3 mg/kg intravenously 5 mg/min up to 20 mg (5–10 mg in adults but may need 20–30 mg), or double this rectally if there is no intravenous access
- midazolam is useful in patients unresponsive to full loading doses of lorazepam, phenobarbital and phenytoin; give a midazolam bolus of 5–15 mg followed by maximal infusion rates of 0.9–11 mg/kg/min.

■ Phenytoin 20 mg/kg intravenously 50 mg/min. Do not exceed 1 g in adults; mix with saline 0.9% (50 ml/500 mg in adults); use in-line filter. Monitor for QT prolongation and stop infusion if it increases by >50% (risk of torsades de pointes).

■ Barbiturate coma: Phenobarbital 20 mg/kg intravenously (maximum 25–30 mg/kg) at 25–50 mg/min; may be given intramuscularly.

Conclusion

Seizures are an infrequent but potentially harmful complication in patients with advanced cancer. Immediate and adequate treatment should be initiated to prevent further insults and preserve quality of life.

Brain metastases

Introduction

Brain metastases are found in 10–30% of cancer patients, and two-thirds of these develop symptoms. The risk of brain metastases is highest in patients with lung cancer (20–40%), breast cancer (10–20%) and malignant melanoma (12–20%). The incidence of brain metastases is rising as a result of advances in imaging procedures and improvements in therapy, which leaves more cancer patients at risk as survival increases.

Symptoms

Brain metastases may cause signs and symptoms due to their localization or to the development of increased intracranial pressure (Table 13.3). The presence of brain metastases should be suspected in all cancer patients who develop neurological symptoms. Progressive neurological dysfunction is usually related to a gradually expanding tumor mass and associated edema or to development of obstructive hydrocephalus. Patients may complain of headache, cognitive disturbances, altered mental status and focal weakness, or nausea and vomiting.

Table 13.3 *Symptoms of brain metastasis*

Symptom	Incidence (%)
Headache	35–50
Nausea/vomiting	30–40
Asthenia	35–40
Seizure	15–20
Dizziness	10–20
Ataxia	15–20
Aphasia	15–20

Diagnosis

- Clinical examination may show focal neurological signs such as aphasia, hemiplegia, hemisensory loss, visual abnormalities and seizures. Other signs are meningismus, papillary eye edema, pupillary and eye movement abnormalities, hypertension, and bradycardia. Patients may lose consciousness.
- Diagnosis is made by CT scan or MRI. MRI is more sensitive than CT scan and facilitates early detection of brain metastases.

Treatment

In patients with advanced cancer, treatment decisions depend on:

- the type of cancer and its sensitivity to radiotherapy or chemotherapy
- the neurological status of the patient
- the extent of systemic disease and its associated symptoms and expected quality of life

Treatment may be etiological, but all patients should receive symptomatic treatment:

- Corticosteroids: dexamethasone 4×4 mg/day orally or higher in case of signs of raised cranial pressure. The dose should be tapered to minimum required doses for symptom control.
- If neurological deficit recovers, consider radiotherapy. Whole-brain radiotherapy associated with supportive care remains the standard treatment for all patients with multiple symptomatic brain metastases or with an isolated symptomatic brain metastasis in the presence of uncontrolled extracranial disease.

- Chemotherapy represents the optimal starting therapy in chemosensitive tumors in patients with asymptomatic multiple or isolated brain metastases and disseminated disease.
- Surgery followed by whole-brain radiotherapy may be indicated in patients with controlled extracranial disease, good performance status and isolated brain metastasis.

Prognosis

The prognosis of patients with brain metastases is determined by the age and general condition of the patient and by the presence of uncontrolled extracranial disease.

In patients with a Karnofsky performance score ≥70%, age under 65 years and controlled extracranial disease, the median survival is 7.1 months; if the age is more than 65 years and there is uncontrolled extracranial disease, the median survival is only 4.2 months, and if the performance score is <70%, the median survival drops to 2.3 months.

Leptomeningeal carcinomatosis

Introduction

Leptomeningeal carcinomatosis is a serious complication of cancer, with substantial morbidity and mortality. The leptomeninges consist of the arachnoid and the pia mater; the space between the two contains the cerebrospinal fluid (CSF). When tumor cells enter the CSF either by direct extension, as in primary brain tumors, or by hematogenous dissemination, they are transported throughout the nervous system by CSF flow, causing either multifocal or diffuse infiltration of the leptomeninges in a sheetlike fashion along the surface of the brain and spinal cord.

Approximately 1–8% of patients with cancer develop leptomeningeal carcinomatosis. The most frequent primary tumors are in the lung (30–70%), breast (10–30%) and gastrointestinal tract (2–20%), or are malignant melanomas (2–15%).

Without therapy, most patients survive for 4–6 weeks, with death occurring because of progressive neurological dysfunction. With therapy, most patients die from systemic complications of their cancer rather than neurological complications of leptomeningeal carcinomatosis. Fixed focal neurological deficits do not improve, but encephalopathies can improve dramatically with treatment.

Symptoms

Meningeal symptoms are the first manifestations in some patients, but most patients already have widespread and progressive cancer with few therapeutic options left. Symptoms include headache (usually associated with nausea, vomiting and lightheadedness), mild gait difficulties from weakness or ataxia, memory problems, incontinence, and sensory abnormalities. Pain and seizures are the most common presenting symptoms.

Diagnosis

- Clinical examination:
  - Cerebral involvement causes headache, lethargy, papillary eye edema, behavior changes and gait disturbance.
  - Cranial nerve involvement causes impaired vision, diplopia (most common), hearing loss and sensory deficits, including vertigo. Palsies of cranial nerves III, V and VI are most common. Cranial nerve deficits are the most frequent signs, presenting in 94% of patients.
  - Spinal root involvement causes meningeal irritation, presenting with nuchal rigidity and neck and back pain, or invasion of the spinal roots. The latter causes leg weakness, radiculopathy (usually lumbar, mimicking a herniated disk), reflex asymmetry or loss, sphincter incontinence, positive Babinski reflexes, paresthesia, and numbness.
- Laboratory tests: CSF examination after gadolinium-enhanced MRI: diagnosis is made with a positive cytology; CSF protein is elevated.
- Imaging studies:
  - Gadolinium-enhanced MRI is the imaging technique of choice and is slightly more sensitive than a CT scan.
  - Myelography, although seldom indicated, may show nodularities or thickening of the nerve roots in approximately 25% of patients.

Treatment

Treatment goals include improvement or stabilization of the patient's neurological status and prolongation of survival. Patients most likely to benefit from therapy are those with indolent systemic cancers that are likely to respond to therapy and those with minimal or absent systemic disease and no fixed neurological deficits.

The intensity of treatment is decided by:

- the presence of a systemic cancer that is responsive to treatment
- preexisting neurological damage and relatively preserved functionality.

Radiation provides palliation of local symptoms. Intrathecal chemotherapy treats subclinical leptomeningeal deposits and tumor cells floating in the CSF, preventing further seeding. The chemotherapeutic agents used are:

- Methotrexate 7 mg/m^2 (usually 12 mg) twice a week for 4 weeks or until CSF clears (persists for 48 hours in CSF), and then weekly or monthly as maintenance therapy; systemic administration may also be effective.
- Cytarabine (cytosine arabinoside, Ara-C) (30 mg/m^2 every day for 3 days) if methotrexate is not tolerated or ineffective; it is not effective for solid tumors, but is useful in leukemic and lymphomatous meningitis. For patients who respond well to treatment, radiation to bulky tumors and symptomatic sites should be started.

Patients who are classified as at high risk may be offered radiotherapy to symptomatic sites or supportive measures only (e.g. analgesics, anticonvulsants or corticosteroids).

Prognosis

Prognosis is generally poor, with the exception of leukemic or lympho-matous meningitis, which is sensitive to both methotrexate and cytarabine, and often can be eradicated completely from the central nervous system.

Among patients with solid tumors, the best response to chemotherapy and radiation occurs in patients with breast cancer, with 60% improving or stabilizing and a median survival of 7 months; 15% survive for 1 year. Only 40% of patients with small-cell lung carcinoma improve or stabilize, and the median survival in these patients is only 4 months. Patients with malignant melanoma have a median survival of 3.6 months, and only 20% of these patients stabilize or improve with treatment.

Non-responders to chemotherapy seldom survive longer than a month.

The most useful prognostic indicator is the Karnofsky performance (KP) score: patients with a KP score ≥70% survive for a mean of 313 days, while those with a KP score ≤60% survive for a mean of only 36 days.

Paraneoplastic neurological syndromes
Introduction

Paraneoplastic neurological syndromes (PNS) are defined as neurological syndromes associated with cancer (Table 13.4). Many of these syndromes are associated with antibodies against neural antigens expressed by the tumor (onconeural antibodies), suggesting that some paraneoplastic neurological symptoms are immune-mediated. The detection of onconeural antibodies has been extremely useful in defining a given neurological syndrome as paraneoplastic. However, PNS may occur without onconeural antibodies, and the antibodies can occur without a neurological syndrome.

PNS are very rare events in patients with cancer, affecting less than 1% of patients.

Symptoms

Neurological symptoms develop acutely and are severe. The clinical course is independent of the cancer's clinical course, and remission of symptoms may occur when the primary tumor is treated. Spontaneous remissions occur, but symptoms are usually irreversible.

■ Patients with encephalomyelitis have a relevant clinical dysfunction at multiple levels of the CNS including the dorsal root ganglia or myenteric plexus. In these patients, where there is prominent dysfunction of a single level of the nervous system, the disorder is described according to the focal syndrome that best includes the signs and symptoms:

  – Limbic encephalitis is clinically suggested by an subacute onset in days or up to 12 weeks of seizures, short-term memory loss, confusion and psychiatric symptoms suggesting involvement of the limbic system.

  – Subacute cerebellar degeneration develops in less than 12 weeks, with a severe pancerebellar syndrome and no MRI evidence of cerebellar atrophy other than that expected from the age of the patient. Symptoms interfere significantly with lifestyle or prevent totally independent existence. Predominant or isolated gait ataxia may be present, but clinical evidence of truncal and hemispheric cerebellar dysfunction is required for the diagnosis.

  – Sensory neuronopathy describes a neurological syndrome characterized by primary damage to the nerve cell body with subacute onset of numbness, and often pain, marked asymmetry of symptoms at onset, involvement of the arms, proprioceptive loss in the areas affected, and electrophysiological studies that show marked, but not restricted, involvement of the sensory fibers with absent sensory nerve action potentials in at least one of the nerves studied.

Table 13.4 Paraneoplastic neurological syndromes

Syndromes of the central nervous system
Encephalomyelitis
Limbic encephalitis
Brainstem encephalitis
Subacute cerebellar degeneration
Opsoclonus–myoclonus
Optic neuritis
Cancer-associated retinopathy
Melanoma-associated retinopathy
Stiff-person syndrome
Necrotizing myelopathy
Motor neuron disease
Syndromes of the peripheral nervous system
Subacute sensory neuronopathy
Acute sensorimotor neuropathy
Guillain–Barré syndrome
Brachial neuritis
Subacute/chronic sensorimotor neuropathies
Neuropathy and paraproteinemia
Neuropathy with vasculitis
Autonomic neuropathy
Chronic gastrointestinal pseudo-obstruction
Acute pandysautonomia
Syndromes of the neuromuscular junction and muscle
Myasthenia gravis
Lambert–Eaton myasthenic syndrome
Acquired neuromyotonia
Dermatomyositis
Acute necrotizing myopathy

- Patients may present with autonomic failure (usually manifested as orthostatic hypotension).
- The clinical course is usually subacutely progressive (lasting for weeks), leading to a bedridden condition if untreated, often in spite of treatment.
- Spontaneous pain is a common symptom with no apparent cause or recognizable distribution.
- Cerebellar dysfunction, encephalomyeloneuropathy and gastrointestinal dysmotility may occur

Diagnosis

- Physical findings in patients with PNS resemble those of any patient with autonomic dysfunction and include the following:
  - orthostatic hypotension in the absence of volume depletion
  - impaired pupillary light responses
  - absence of heart rate changes with respiration
  - abnormal Valsalva response
  - abnormal cold pressor response
  - impotence
  - peripheral sensory neuronopathy, which is often evident as patchy superficial sensory loss and asymmetrically abnormal stretch reflexes. Patchy asymmetric weakness and dyscoordination or abnormal mental status may occur in patients with CNS involvement.
- Onconeural antibodies (Table 13.5): serum analysis for the presence of antineuronal autoantibodies by immunohistochemistry and immunoblotting is the key to diagnosis.
- Lumbar puncture is often necessary for cytological analysis in addition to the other usual tests.
- Electromyogram (EMG)/nerve conduction velocity (NCV) studies can confirm the patchy nature of deficits, abnormal autonomic skin responses and denervation of muscle due to motor neuron involvement.
- Imaging studies: since patients with PNS often have more widespread neurological abnormalities, and the underlying primary is often small-cell lung cancer, brain MRI scanning is appropriate to detect metastases.

Treatment

Treatment of patients with PNS depends on severity of failure and status of the associated malignancy.

Table 13.5 Onconeural antibodies

Antibody	Paraneoplastic neurological syndrome	Tumors
Anti-Hu (ANNA1)	Encephalomyelitis, sensory neuronopathy, chronic gastrointestinal pseudo-obstruction; paraneoplastic cerebellar degeneration, limbic encephalitis	SCLC
Anti-Yo (PCA1)	Paraneoplastic cerebellar degeneration	Ovary, breast
Anti-CV2 (CRMP5)	Encephalomyelitis, chorea, sensory neuronopathy, sensorimotor neuropathy; chronic gastrointestinal pseudo-obstruction; paraneoplastic cerebellar degeneration, limbic encephalitis	SCLC, thymoma
Anti-Ri (ANNA2)	Brainstem encephalitis	Breast, SCLC
Anti-Ma2	Limbic/diencephalic encephalitis, brainstem encephalitis, paraneoplastic cerebellar degeneration	Testicular Lung
Anti-amphiphysin	Stiff-person syndrome, various syndromes	Breast, SCLC

SCLC, small cell lung cancer.

125

- Autonomic failure
  - The most disabling symptom is often orthostatic hypotension, which may respond to pressors (e.g. ephedrine, phenylpropanolamine, caffeine) and volume expansion (fludrocortisone and salt). In severe cases, consider compressive clothing.
  - Laxatives and other bowel care may be needed to treat gastrointestinal motility disorders.
  - Bladder dysfunction may require the administration of bethanechol or catheterization.
- Autoimmune process: no therapy to suppress the autoimmune response has been shown to be reliably effective; however, successful treatment of the associated malignancy by surgery and/or chemotherapy may slow or stop the progression of the neurological syndrome.

Paraneoplastic syndromes with muscle rigidity

Stiff-person syndrome is characterized by progressive muscle rigidity, stiffness and painful spasms triggered by auditory, sensory or emotional stimuli. Rigidity mainly involves the lower trunk and legs, but it can affect the upper extremities and neck. Symptoms improve with sleep and general anesthesia.

Stiff-person syndrome has been reported in association with breast cancer, Hodgkin's disease and colon cancer.

Paraneoplastic stiff-person syndrome is associated with antibodies against amphiphysin, a synaptic protein involved in vesicle endocytosis. Antibodies against glutamic acid decarboxylase have also been reported, and some patients have antibodies to both amphiphysin and glutamic acid decarboxylase.

Optimal treatment of stiff-person syndrome requires therapy of the underlying tumor, glucocorticoids and symptomatic use of drugs that enhance γ-aminobutyric acid (GABA)-ergic transmission (diazepam, baclofen and valproic acid).

Paraneoplastic neuromyotonia is a syndrome of spontaneous and continuous muscle fiber activity of peripheral origin. Unlike stiff-person syndrome, this abnormal activity persists during sleep.

The disorder frequently develops in association with myasthenia gravis (MG) in thymoma. Hodgkin's disease, plasma cell dyscrasia and small-cell lung cancer have been associated with neuromyotonia.

Autoantibodies against voltage-gated potassium channels have been found in some patients with paraneoplastic neuromyotonia.

The disorder may improve spontaneously or with plasmapheresis. Whether antineoplastic treatment benefits these patients in general is unclear.

Neuromuscular junction disorder

Introduction

Lambert–Eaton myasthenic syndrome (LEMS) is a presynaptic disorder of the neuromuscular junction that can cause weakness similar to that of myasthenia gravis (MG). Typical MG is associated with thymoma in approximately 15% of patients. In approximately 60% of patients with LES, the disorder is associated with an underlying cancer, usually small cell lung carcinoma.

Symptoms

The proximal muscles of the lower limbs are most commonly affected. Cranial nerve findings, including ptosis of the eyelids and diplopia, occur in up to 70% of patients and resemble features of MG. In contrast to MG, patients with LEMS have depressed or absent reflexes, show autonomic changes such as dry mouth and impotence, and show incremental rather than decremental responses on repetitive nerve stimulation.

Diagnosis

LEMS is caused by autoantibodies directed against P/Q-type calcium channels at the motor nerve terminals, which can be detected in about 85% of LEMS patients by radioimmunoassay. These antibodies block acetylcholine release from nerve terminals.

Treatment

Most patients with LES benefit from plasmapheresis and immunosuppressive therapy. Drugs that increase presynaptic acetylcholine release may also decrease symptoms; 3,4-diaminopyridine is one such agent that has relatively minimal side effects.

Cranial neuropathies

Introduction

The frequency of metastatic disease causing cranial and peripheral nerve dysfunction is unknown because only a few studies have addressed this issue. Microscopic ocular metastases have been found in 12.6% of patients who died of cancer. Facial nerve paralysis occurs in 5–25% of malignant parotid neoplasms.

Metastatic lesions may affect cranial nerves at any point. Tumors can affect cranial nerves either by compression without directly breaching the epineurium or by invasion along perineural and endoneural planes. Metastases to the base of the skull (e.g. breast and lung cancers) often cause cranial nerve dysfunction.

Leptomeningeal metastases, an increasingly common complication of cancer (e.g. lymphoma and breast cancer), may cause multiple cranial neuropathies.

Brain stem metastases occasionally cause isolated cranial nerve dysfunction, especially of the sixth cranial nerve.

Cranial neuropathies also occur as side effects of treatment (radio- and/or chemotherapy) or as paraneoplastic syndromes (Table 13.6).

Diagnosis

■ In the case of clinical suspicion, MRI is performed for the evaluation of the cranial nerve along its entire course.
■ CT scan is indicated when skull base invasion is suspected.
■ Lumbar puncture should be performed in the evaluation of cranial neuropathies, especially when multiple cranial nerves are affected.

Treatment

■ Radiotherapy is indicated for skull base and orbital metastases.
■ Chemotherapy is indicated for chemosensitive cancers (e.g. lymphoma).

Table 13.6 Nonmetastatic causes of cranial neuropathy in cancer patients

Cranial nerve (symptoms)	Causes
III (diplopia, ptosis)	Increased intracranial pressure, paraneoplastic myasthenia gravis
IV (diplopia)	Vincristine
VI (diplopia)	Vincristine, increased intracranial pressure
VIII (hearing loss)	Cisplatin, radiotherapy-induced serous otitis
X (laryngeal paralysis)	Vincristine

Plexopathy

Introduction

Plexopathy is an uncommon though not rare cause of pain in cancer patients, and it may mimic symptoms of many common neuropathies. Lesions of the plexus may be secondary to cancer that reaches the plexus by direct extension or by metastasis through lymphatics or previous radiotherapy.

The cervical, brachial and lumbosacral plexus may be involved. Breast and lung cancer (Pancoast's tumor) cause brachial plexopathy, pelvic malignancies cause lumbosacral plexopathy,and cancer of the head and neck or cervical lymph nodes causes cervical plexopathy.

Symptoms

Pain is the most common symptom in patients with plexopathy. Pain may precede other symptoms by weeks or months. Patients may complain of numbness, paresthesia, allodynia, hyperesthesia, weakness or edema.

In brachial plexopathy, pain is the initial symptom, arising in the shoulder and radiating down the medial aspect of the arm, elbow and forearm to the fourth and fifth fingers. In Pancoast's syndrome, ipsilateral Horner's syndrome (ptosis, miosis and anhydrosis) is also present and is due to stellate ganglion invasion by the tumor.

Differential diagnosis

The differential diagnosis includes radiation-induced plexopathy, trauma and idiopathic plexopathy. The initial symptom is pain in metastatic plexopathy and paresthesia in radiation-induced plexopathy. Horner's syndrome is present in metastatic but is not seen in radiation-induced plexopathy. Rapid progression of the symptoms also favors metastatic plexopathy.

It is important to distinguish between lumbosacral plexopathy and the cauda equina syndrome resulting from epidural or meningeal metastases. Bilateral involvement is usually a sign of cauda equina involvement, but may be seen in some metastatic plexopathies. In addition to the cauda equina syndrome, the differential diagnosis includes herniated lumbar disk, radiation-induced plexopathy, trauma, diabetes and idiopathic lumbosacral plexopathy.

Diagnosis

■ Physical examination findings depend on the specific parts of the plexus involved. Weakness and sensory loss in certain dermatomes may be present. More widespread involvement may lead to motor and sensory loss. Less common primary cancers may occur and present as limb pain and/or a tender mass, causing radiating paresthesia upon palpation. Sensory and motor deficits may be found corresponding to the tumor's location in the plexus.

- Laboratory studies: a general laboratory survey with a complete metabolic panel, vitamin B12 and folic acid, complete blood count, and urinalysis should be performed. Also to be considered are tumor markers (e.g. carcinoembryonic antigen (CEA) in a patient with prior colon cancer, prostate-specific antigen (PSA) in a patient with prior prostate cancer) and serum protein electrophoresis.

- Imaging studies:
  - Plain radiographs should be obtained to look for neoplastic changes.
  - MRI of the plexus has a high sensitivity in detecting cancer involvement of the plexus; however, both CT scan and MRI can present difficulty in detecting infiltrating cancer and distinguishing it from radiation fibrosis. A well-defined mass lesion on CT scans or MRI is more suggestive of tumor-induced than radiotherapy-induced plexopathy.
  - Bone scan may be helpful to detect metastases.
  - Positron emission tomography (PET) may be useful in identifying metastases in or near the plexus.

- Nerve conduction and electromyography studies: in general, electrodiagnostic examination is used to localize a lesion, characterize its pathology, establish a prognosis and facilitate a treatment plan. The key question is whether the limb weakness is due to axonometic (dead) or neurapraxic (functionally blocked) axons.
  - Nerve conduction studies may reveal axon loss that is often so severe that lower trunk-mediated sensory potentials are absent, and motor responses are of low amplitude or absent. Needle examination often reveals motor unit potential loss and spontaneous activity.
  - Comparison of the amplitude of a peripheral evoked response after 7 days with that of the contralateral side can provide an estimate of the degree of injury/recovery. Despite the potential utility of electrodiagnostic studies, limitations exist. When pain is the only initial symptom, EMG results may be within the reference range, although the results almost always reveal abnormalities by the time permanent motor and/or sensory deficits are present.
  - Somatosensory evoked potentials (SSEP) are noninvasive tests that may be used to assess sensory impairments associated with plexopathy.

Treatment

Treatment of plexopathy should be interdisciplinary, including medication and prescription of physical, occupational and recreational therapies. Treatment is often difficult and palliative. In patients with tumor-induced plexopathy, chemotherapy and radiotherapy (up to 50% of patients obtain significant pain relief) are used if the tumor is sensitive.

Adequate pain control is the most important goal.

No medications are specific for the treatment of plexopathy. Typical analgesic and adjunct analgesic agents may be worthwhile in managing neoplastic plexopathy. Opiates may be effective at acceptable doses and often are tried first.

Nonsteroidal anti-inflammatory drugs can be helpful and are usually tried in combination with other agents. Adjunct agents such as tricyclic antidepressants (e.g. amitriptyline), and anticonvulsants (valproic acid) may be used to control neuropathic pain.

Paravertebral nerve blocks may be indicated, depending on the location of the tumor. However, plexopathy is often widespread and not amenable to the application of selective blocks.

Further reading

Arnold SM, Lieberman FS, Foon KA: Paraneoplastic syndromes. In: De Vita VT Jr, Hellman S, Rosenberg SA (eds), Cancer: Principles and Practice of Oncology, 7th edn. Philadelphia: Lippincott Williams & Wilkins, 2005: 2200–07.

Caraceni A, Martini C, Simonetti F: Neurological problems in advanced cancer. In: Doyle D, Hanks G, Cherny NI (eds), Oxford Textbook of Palliative Medicine, 3rd edn. Oxford: Oxford University Press, 2004: 702–30.

Chang EL, Lo S: Diagnosis and management of central nervous system metastases from breast cancer. Oncologist 2003; 8: 398–410.

Dalmau J, Rosenfeld MR: Paraneoplastic neurologic syndromes. In: Kasper DL, Braunwald E, Fauci AS et al (eds), Harrison's Principles of Internal Medicine, 16th edn. New York: McGraw-Hill, 2005: 571–5.

DeAngelis LM, Posner JB: Neurologic complications. In: Kufe DW, Pollock RE, Weichselbaum RR et al (eds), Holland–Frei Cancer Medicine, 6th edn. Hamilton, Canada: BC Decker, 2003: 2451–68.

Graus F, Delattre JY, Antoine JC: Recommended diagnostic criteria for paraneoplastic neurological syndromes. J Neurol Neurosurg Psychiatry 2004; 75: 1135–40.

Posner JB: Neurologic Complications of Cancer. Philadelphia: FA Davis, 1995.

Psychiatric problems

F Stiefel, D Stagno
Service de Psychiatrie de Liaison, University Hospital
Lausanne, Switzerland

Introduction

The prevalence rate of psychiatric disorders in cancer patients is estimated to be as high as 50%, which is approximately twice the prevalence reported for psychiatric disorders in medical patients and three times the estimate for the general population. Most of these disorders are considered to be highly treatable. Unfortunately, the assumption that emotional distress is just a foreseeable and ordinary reaction to cancer has long prevented the accurate assessment and treatment of psychiatric disorders in the cancer population. In the meantime, several studies have indicated that psychological distress can have serious negative consequences for patients with advanced cancer or terminally ill cancer patients, including reduced quality of life, severe suffering and a desire for hastened death, request for physician-assisted suicide, suicide, and psychological distress in family and staff members.

Adjustment disorders
Definition and prevalence

Adjustment disorders are defined as an inability to cope with or a maladaptive reaction to one or several identifiable stressful life event(s)/stressor(s) (e.g. divorce, family crises or physical illness). Symptoms of anxious and depressed mood interfering with social functioning occur within 3 months of the stressor(s), persist for no longer than 6 months, and seem in excess of what would be normally expected.

In 1983, Derogatis et al reported the prevalence of psychiatric disorders in a cohort of randomly accessed cancer in- and outpatients. By *Diagnostic and Statistical Manual of Mental Disorders* (3rd edition) (DSM-III) criteria, 53% showed no psychiatric disorder, revealing a proper adjustment to cancer-related stress. However, 47% of that sample met the criteria for a DSM-III disorder. Among them, 68% were diagnosed with an adjustment disorder.

Etiology and differential diagnoses

Adjustment disorders are thought to arise as a direct consequence of stress or trauma. The clinical manifestations include depressed mood, anxiety, feeling of inability to cope, loss of control and low self-esteem. Hospitalization, illness, investigations and treatment may produce adjustment disorders. Moreover, stressors not related to medical problems, such as family problems or professional or financial difficulties, can contribute to the development of an adjustment disorder.

■ Adjustment disorders should be distinguished from acute stress reactions, which are transient disorders that subside within hours or days. Such symptoms usually appear within minutes of the impact of the stressful event (e.g. cancer diagnosis or relapse). Cognitive impairment, with attention deficit, daze, numbness and comprehension difficulties, is present at first, and is followed by behavioral symptoms such as agitation, withdrawal and anxiety.

■ Adjustment disorders should also be distinguished from post-traumatic stress disorder (PTSD), which occurs as a delayed response to a stressful event. Typical symptoms include episodes of repeated reliving of the trauma in intrusive memories, visions and nightmares, and avoidance of activities and situations that may recall the original trauma. They may also be associated with outbursts of fear, panic, aggression, anxiety and depression. In most publications, prevalence rates of PTSD among cancer patients range from 5% to 22%, which is a little below the estimates for the general population (9–24%), suggesting that cancer would be no more severe or traumatic in itself than other stress factors in everyday life.

■ Bereavement is a normal reaction to loss, and usually decreases over time. Feelings of sadness, despair or helplessness are associated with a preserved capacity to relate to others and with socially occupationally normal functioning. A mourning person still experiences life as worth living and is perceived by him/herself and others as coherent and essentially unchanged with regard to personality and way of coping.

■ Adjustment disorders should not be confused with other mood disorders such as major or minor depression, dysthymia, generalized anxiety disorder or panic disorder.

A specific adjustment disorder in cancer is anticipatory nausea and vomiting. Some patients during the course of chemotherapy experience several symptoms that precede the treatment: nausea and vomiting (conditioned symptoms), often associated with anxiety, depression and helplessness.

Chemotherapy can therefore be considered as a major stressor, and any treatment able to prevent such a condition should be employed.

Diagnostic procedures

The medical interview is the best way of establishing a diagnosis of adjustment disorder and making a therapeutic alliance with the patient. However, standardized interviews by well-trained health-care professionals are expensive and very demanding in human resources. It is therefore more convenient to utilize screening tools for general psychopathology. Among the screening instruments, the best studied are the self-administered questionnaires: Beck's Depression Inventory, Zung's Self-Rating Depression Scale, the General Health Questionnaire, the Brief Symptom Inventory, the Edinburgh Depression Scale, and the Hospital Anxiety and Depression Scale (HADS). They usually take less than 15 minutes to complete and have proven to be acceptable to most patients and clinicians.

The determination of the optimal cutoff point is a major issue for screening instruments. For example, several studies screening for psychological distress in cancer patients with the Hospital Anxiety and Depression Scale suggest a cutoff point between 10 and 11 for adjustment disorder and a cutoff point between 17 and 19 for major depression.

Research efforts are mainly focused on the evaluation of anxiety and depression, the most frequent symptoms of adjustment disorders in the medically ill, especially in palliative settings. Their purpose is to improve the quality of life, the compliance and the satisfaction of palliative care patients, whose psychological problems are still underdiagnosed and underrated.

Treatment

Although treatment options constantly overlap in clinical practice, they can be schematically divided into two categories, like most psychiatric disorders: psychological interventions and pharmacotherapy.

Psychological interventions

■ Providing information is the first step in helping patients cope with cancer. However, information on diagnosis, prognosis, treatments and long-term consequences may be distorted by psychological factors, especially in the case of bad news. Information, therefore, must be repeated several times and adapted to patients' needs.

■ Counseling is a special form of help performed by nurses, social workers or volunteers whose purpose is to help patients to express and understand their feelings about cancer and encourage them to cope with the situation. Although such interventions are not well formalized, several meta-analyses have witnessed their efficacy in promoting a sense of control and reducing depressive symptoms or anxiety. Counseling is a first-line support where no specialized treatment is required.

■ Psychotherapy is based on the development of a trusting relationship that allows free communication between patient and therapist. Every type of psychotherapy is defined by the use of specific techniques depending on theoretical backgrounds. Schematically, psychotherapies for cancer patients can be divided into the psychodynamic psychotherapies and cognitive–behavioral treatments.

  – Behavioral therapies are based on conditioning theories. They involve precise observation of behavior and use directive methods to achieve determined goals. The positive effects of behavioral techniques are documented by controlled studies. Behavioral therapies are formalized, and the training of specialists, as well as research efforts, are organized. Nevertheless, none of them has offered sound evidence of major efficacy. Their strength (and limitation) is that they are symptom-centered. For example, they have proven effective in treating anticipatory nausea and vomiting associated with chemotherapy or postprostatectomy urinary incontinence. Behavioral treatments have been proposed to relieve cancer-related symptoms in the palliative setting and are considered to be useful in the treatment of dyspnea in the terminally ill. Techniques consist of hypnosis, relaxation, progressive muscle relaxation training, imagery, and systematic desensitization. Cognitive therapies deal with maladaptive thoughts, irrational beliefs and other psychological factors responsible for psychological or somatic symptoms. These thoughts are confronted with reason and reality, thus promoting a better adjustment, for example, in the terminally ill with adjustment disorder or major depression.

  – Two models of psychodynamic psychotherapy are used with cancer patients: supportive and dynamic psychotherapies.

  (1) In supportive psychotherapy, the therapist's goal is to activate the residual resources of a patient in order to restore balance and a sense of self-confidence.

  (2) Dynamic psychotherapy, based on the psychoanalytical model, suggests that unconscious conflicts are responsible for a large part of the psychological problems.

In general, dynamic psychotherapies, because of their complexity and the specificity of their goals, seem to be inappropriate to treat the physically ill and especially terminally ill cancer patients. Nevertheless, new short-term models are promising; they will possibly support the clinical experience suggesting that dynamic psychotherapy is effective in the cancer setting.

Pharmacotherapy

In clinical practice, it has been observed than over half of cancer patients receive psychotropic medication, mainly prescribed by the oncologist or the general practitioner; most of these patients are on minor tranquilizers, half of them are on antidepressants, and more than a third receive at least two drugs. In adjustment disorders, the medication is intended to treat depressive and anxious symptoms. These treatments are described in the sections below.

Anxiety

Definition and prevalence

Anxiety can be classified according to DSM-V. These definitions are useful for research purposes, but not for daily clinical work, because anxiety in palliative patients may be caused by different events and factors than in the general psychiatric population. In a recent study including more than 700 patients, anxiety was diagnosed in 13% of the patients, by HADS. Not all anxious states, however, are pathological or clinically relevant. Anxiety serves as a physiological reaction to signal danger to human beings and is, in a way, part of every physical illness. In terminally ill patients, the recognition of anxious symptoms requiring treatment can therefore be challenging.

Clinical presentation and etiology

Patients with anxiety complain of tension or restlessness, or they exhibit jitteriness, autonomic hyperactivity, hypervigilance, insomnia, distractibility, shortness of breath, numbness, apprehension, worry or rumination. Often the physical manifestations of anxiety overshadow the psychological or cognitive ones. The assumption that a high level of anxiety is inevitably encountered during the terminal phase of cancer is neither helpful nor accurate. In deciding whether to treat anxiety in the terminally ill, a patient's subjective level of distress is the primary criterion for the initiation of a treatment. Other considerations include problematic patient behavior, such as noncompliance due to anxiety, family's and caregivers' discomfort at a patient's distress, and the balance between the risks and benefits of treatment.

Anxiety may be encountered as a component of an adjustment disorder, panic disorder, PTSD, phobic disorder, generalized anxiety disorder or agitated depression. In terminally ill cancer patients, anxiety often arises from illness- or treatment-related complications. Hypoxia, metabolic disorders (e.g. hypercalcemia), sepsis, uncontrolled pain, and adverse drug reactions (e.g. corticosteroids or opioids) or withdrawal syndromes (with alcohol or benzodiazepines) often present as anxiety. Anxiety is also a prominent symptom of delirium; up to 50% of delirious patients report anxiety as one of the major symptoms. Even though anxiety is frequently the manifestation of somatic complications in the terminally ill, it is important to remember that psychological factors related to death and dying or existential issues may play a role in anxiety, particularly in alert, not confused patients. Anxious states that have a spiritual and existential dimension illustrate the fact that anxiety is not the exclusive domain of medicine.

Diagnosis

The clinical interview with the patient and family remains the best approach to assess anxiety; such interventions often have a therapeutic effect, since patients are invited to express their feelings in a containing environment. Several of the screening instruments mentioned in the adjustment disorders section may also be of help. The main differential diagnosis in the terminally ill is delirium;faced with a restless, apparently alert patient, attention deficit must be accurately sought for, in order not to miss delirium. The assumption that anxiety is quite normal in advanced cancer patients is the principal impediment to an accurate assessment and an effective treatment of anxiety.

Treatment

The pharmacotherapy of anxiety in terminal illness involves the careful use of several classes of drugs: benzodiazepines, typical and atypical neuroleptics, and antidepressants.

■ Benzodiazepines are the most commonly used treatment in this population. The shorter-acting (4–8 hours) benzodiazepines, such as lorazepam, oxazepam and alprazolam, are reasonably safe here. Lorazepam and oxazepam are preferred for patients with liver failure. Alprazolam is metabolized through oxidative pathways in the liver and should be used with caution in cases of severe hepatic damage. Short-acting drugs avoid toxic

138

accumulation due to impaired metabolism and may be indicated in debilitated individuals. Unfortunately, patients often experience breakthrough anxiety or end-of-dose failure with short-acting compounds. Doses are usually lower than those used in the physically healthy population.

■ Neuroleptics, such as haloperidol, methotrimeprazine or thioridazine, or newer drugs, such as olanzapine, risperidone and quetiapine, are useful in the treatment of anxiety when benzodiazepines are not sufficient for symptom control. They are also indicated when an organic etiology is suspected or when psychotic symptoms such as delusions or hallucinations accompany the anxiety. Olanzapine has proven to be efficient in the treatment of anxious or delirious patients. Risperidone and quetiapine offer valid alternatives. There has been a case report of sudden death under low doses of risperidone, which recalls the potential harm of all psychotropics. Extrapyramidal side effects, acute dystonia and neuroleptic malignant syndrome are also potential risks of neuroleptics.

■ Antidepressants are useful in treating anxiety associated with agitated depression.

Depression
Definition and prevalence

Cancer patients are significantly more depressed than members of the general population, with a prevalence of 13–18%. Depression is a significant symptom for approximately one in four palliative care patients and is especially common in those patients with more advanced metastatic disease.

The assessment of depression is generally based on DSM-V criteria.

The standard clinical presentation includes psychological and somatic symptoms: depressed mood, loss of interest, mood changes, hopelessness, helplessness, suicidal ideation, guilt or poor concentration. Frequently observed somatic symptoms are fatigue, insomnia, psychomotor retardation or agitation, and constipation. However, some physical symptoms consistent with depression can also be observed among cancer patients without any mood disturbance.

Consequently, the diagnosis of a major depressive syndrome in terminally ill patients often relies on the psychological or cognitive symptoms of major depression (i.e. feelings of worthlessness, hopelessness and excessive guilt, and suicidal ideation). On the other hand, to rely on the psychological or cognitive signs and symptoms for the assessment of depression in palliative patients is not without problems. Feelings of hopelessness, worthlessness and guilt, or suicidal ideation may appear as logical when there is no cure or when the pain cannot be easily controlled. These feelings deserve to be carefully evaluated and contextualized. Hopelessness that is pervasive and associated with despair is more likely to represent a symptom of depression. Guilt and worthlessness are also ambiguous symptoms. Patients often complain of being a burden for their family and eventually family members are subjected to great pressure by their relative's illness. But excessive guilt and feelings of worthlessness reveal the patient's difficulty in adapting to a new family pattern, where their role and position are challenged by the disease.

Etiology

Depression in cancer patients is often caused by multiple psychological and biological factors.

Psychological factors, such as anticipatory grief over the impending loss of life, loved ones and autonomy, may lead to depression.

On the other hand, the imbalance of several immunological and endocrinal systems is probably implicated in the pathogenesis of depression: for example, circulating proinflammatory cytokines, such as interleukin-1 (IL-1), IL-6 and tumor necrosis factor α (TNF-α), either produced by certain cancers (e.g. pancreatic cancer) or administered as components of immunotherapy protocols, are linked with depression. In animal models, it has been shown that cytokines produce hypersomnia, psychomotor retardation, fatigue, reduced exploratory behavior, cognitive impairment, impaired social behavior, anhedonia, and decreased libido and sexual activity. Among humans, the same behavioral changes have been clinically assessed and grouped in a syndrome called sickness behavior. In cancer patients, cytokines are associated with a high prevalence of depressive disorders, with impaired quality of life.

Other common causes of depression in cancer patients include chronic or uncontrolled pain, medications (e.g. corticosteroids, vincristine or cimetidine), metabolic alterations (e.g. hypercalcemia) and damage to the central nervous system by the tumor or its treatment.

Diagnostic procedures

Clinical evaluation consists of a careful evaluation of the aforementioned symptoms. The differential diagnosis of depression includes sadness, adjustment disorder with depressed mood, grief and delirium. Criteria have been proposed to be used in diagnosing major depressive syndromes in medical patients. Somatic items such as decreased appetite and sleep, fatigue, and complaints about lessened concentration could be replaced by psychological items such as fearfulness or depressed appearance, social withdrawal or decreased talkativeness, brooding self-pity, and pessimism.

Treatment

Once the cause of depression has been established and a causal therapeutic approach (e.g. treatment of hypercalcemia) is not possible, psychotherapy and pharmacotherapy are useful approaches to treat depression in terminally ill patients.

■ The different types of psychotherapy described in the adjustment disorder section may also be applied to patients suffering from major depressive disorders. Supportive short-term psychotherapies are preferred in order to restore coping strategies.

■ Severe depression usually requires combined treatments with psychotropic drugs. There are several psychotropic drugs currently accepted as being effective in oncology, and the efficacy of selective serotonin reuptake inhibitors (SSRI), tricyclic antidepressants (TCAs) and psychostimulants is supported by several studies.

   – Mianserin, a heterocyclic antidepressant with analgesic properties, has shown a superiority over placebo in two blinded randomized controlled trials (RCTs). An RCT with trimipramine in 42 cancer patients with major depression showed improvement in depressive symptoms independently of improvement in physical functioning. Two studies comparing an SSRI and a TCA (fluoxetine vs desipramine, and paroxetine vs amitriptyline) failed to show a major difference between these two classes of drugs in depressive symptoms.

   – In clinical practice, SSRI are preferred to TCAs because they are known to cause fewer adverse reactions.

   – Three studies in cancer patients with depression proved the efficacy of a psychostimulant (methylphenidate), which is a valid alternative when a rapid onset of action is required and when patients cannot tolerate the lethargy and weakness that frequently accompany advanced disease. Psychostimulants are often associated with a significant improvement in cognitive functioning. It should be noted that in recent years, contradictory results have emerged about the possible roles of antidepressants in carcinogenesis.

Fatigue

Definition and prevalence

The National Comprehensive Cancer Network Fatigue Practice Guidelines Panel has defined fatigue as 'An unusual, persistent, subjective sense of tiredness related to cancer or cancer treatment that interferes with usual functioning'. Fatigue is a subjective sensation with physical (e.g. decreased energy), cognitive (e.g. decreased concentration) and affective (e.g. decreased motivation) modes of expression. Cancer-related fatigue criteria have also been proposed by the *International Classification of Diseases* (ICD). Fatigue is the most common symptom associated with cancer and its treatments. Prevalence estimates vary from 60% to 90%. Cancer-related fatigue differs from fatigue in healthy individuals because it occurs despite adequate amounts of rest or sleep. Fatigue can persist for months or years after cancer treatment has been completed. In patients with advanced cancer, fatigue can accompany symptoms of depression, pain, anorexia, insomnia, anxiety, nausea and dyspnea, all of which can contribute to fatigue.

Etiology

In advanced cancer patients, multiple etiological factors for fatigue may coexist.

Tumors can produce proinflammatory cytokines that produce conditions that contribute to fatigue, such as anemia, cachexia, anorexia, fever, infection and depression. Cachexia and anorexia occur in the majority of patients with advanced cancer. The underlying pathogenesis involves metabolic and neurohormonal abnormalities, secondary to immune alterations, including cytokine production. An association between depression and fatigue has been observed, although a causal relationship has not been established. Other possible etiologies are pre-existing comorbidities, endocrine abnormalities, medications (e.g. opioids, anxiolytics, hypnotics, antiemetics, anti-hypertensives, corticosteroids), sleep disorders, pain, nausea and dyspnea.

Diagnostic procedures

Patients should be screened for the presence and severity of fatigue at their first visit with an oncologist and at appropriate intervals thereafter. When screening reveals moderate or severe fatigue, possible etiologic factors should be assessed. For fatigue assessment, the severity, temporal features (onset, course, duration and daily pattern), worsening or relieving factors, associated distress, and impact on daily life must be evaluated. Several fatigue assessment tools exist, but the multidimensional fatigue assessment tools incorporating multiple characteristics of fatigue and their impact on function require a time-consuming administration and are therefore more useful in a research setting.

Treatment

The purpose of treatment measures is to reduce fatigue intensity or help patients function at a stable level of fatigue. Specific interventions target possibly reversible causes of fatigue (e.g. hypothyroidism). When the cause is irreversible and unknown, symptomatic interventions, such as education, counseling and pharmacological measures, can be useful.

■ Exercise is the nonpharmacological intervention with the strongest evidence of therapeutic benefit.
■ Pharmacological treatments are also useful, even if they are not yet supported by well-designed studies.
  – Corticosteroids have been shown to decrease fatigue, when used over a short period of time (prolonged corticosteroid treatment is considered to cause fatigue). Their mechanism of action is unknown.
  – Progestational agents, such as megestrol acetate, are indicated to improve appetite and caloric intake. They have proven to be beneficial on activity levels, with a short onset of action.
  – Methylphenidate is prescribed to treat opioid-induced somnolence, reduce pain intensity, and improve mood and cognition, as well as fatigue.
  – Modafinil is a psychostimulant with potentially fewer side effects than methylphenidate and is currently being studied in the treatment of cancer-related fatigue.
  – Promising treatment options include agents that prevent the release of cytokines (pentoxifylline, thalidomide and bradykinin antagonists) or inhibit cytokine action (i.e. cyclooxygenase-1 and -2 (COX-1 and -2) inhibitors and selective COX-2 inhibitors).

Sleep disorders
Definition and prevalence

Insomnia is a heterogeneous complaint that may involve difficulty in falling asleep (initial or sleep onset insomnia), difficulty in staying asleep with prolonged nocturnal awakenings (middle or maintenance insomnia), early-morning awakening with inability to resume sleep (terminal or late insomnia), or the complaint of nonrestorative sleep. In one study conducted among women with breast cancer, 51% reported insomnia symptoms and 19% met the criteria for insomnia disorder, which is twice as frequent as in the general population. In various studies with cancer patients, sleep problems ranged from 30% to 50% in the cancer population.

Etiology

Risk factors are hyperarousability, female gender (twice the prevalence), aging, and personal or family history of insomnia. In cancer patients, the co-occurrence of another psychiatric disorder is a predisposing factor for insomnia: insomnia is an important symptom of anxiety, depressive disorders and delirium. Insomnia is generally precipitated by stressful life events, such as medical illness. Cancer is characterized by a succession of severe stressors, each of which can precipitate insomnia. Some cancer treatments may increase the risk of developing insomnia, because of their emotional impact, their direct physiological effects or their side effects. Finally, cancer pain is an obvious etiological factor: 60–80% of advanced cancer patients experience pain, and pain affects both the initiation and maintenance of sleep.

Diagnostic procedures

For practical reasons, insomnia is best defined in oncology as a complaint by the patient – similar to the definition of pain – of poor or unsatisfactory sleep; this complaint may include different aspects, such as difficulty in initiating sleep, repeated or lengthy awakenings, early awakening, inadequate total sleep time, poor quality of sleep, or daytime dysfunction, such as change of alertness, loss of energy, or cognitive, behavioral or emotional changes. A clinical interview is the standard approach to assess insomnia. Recently, a diagnostic tool, the Insomnia Severity Index (ISI), has been valididated in the cancer population. The ISI includes seven items using Likert-type scales to evaluate the perceived severity of insomnia during the last 2 weeks. It seems to be an effective screening tool in the context of cancer, and, given the fact that it takes only 5 minutes to complete and is easy to score, it could be implemented in oncology.

The first step with a cancer patient complaining of insomnia should be an accurate evaluation of the reported symptoms. While this may be considered common sense, it must be recalled that 53% of physicians evaluating elderly patients neglect to elicit any sleep history.

An accurate evaluation includes diagnosis, identification of precipitating factors, and assessment of maladaptive cognitive, behavioral and emotional responses to insomnia. An adequate sleep history, including sleep and wakefulness patterns, history of the bed partner, family history of sleep disorders and previous treatments, should be obtained. Complaints of inadequate sleep in the absence of any residual daytime effects or distress do not indicate significant insomnia.

Insomnia causes psychosocial, physical and occupational disturbances, commonly reported as fatigue/lethargy, mood disturbances, cognitive inefficiency, motor impairments, social discomfort and nonspecific physical symptoms. Physiological and health consequences are of particular importance in the context of cancer: sleep disturbance is associated with increased pain perception, increased mortality and deleterious effects on immune functioning.

Treatment

The initial strategy is to treat underlying physical and psychological factors contributing to sleep disturbances. It is essential, for instance, to manage pain or delirium with appropriate treatments, before focusing on insomnia with pharmacological or psychological approaches.

Pharmacotherapy

Hypnotic medications are the most commonly used treatment for insomnia. They include some benzodiazepines and newer nonbenzodiazepine hypnotics (zolpidem, zopiclon and zaleplon), which are believed to have more specific hypnotic effects and less residual effects the next day. Benzodiazepines can cause delirium, especially in the elderly, and produce excessive sedation, especially when associated with opiates. Some antidepressant drugs, predominantly those with sedative properties such as mirtazapine (15 mg), can be useful in the treatment of insomnia, especially in depressed patients.

Psychological treatments

According to the cognitive–behavioral conceptualization of insomnia, maladaptive sleep habits and dysfunctional cognitions are the most important factors maintaining insomnia. These maladaptative sleep behaviors are particularly frequent in cancer patients who are encouraged to get rest and sleep to recuperate from their cancer treatments. Several interventions, such as stimulus control, sleep restriction or relaxation, have been used successfully for the treatment of insomnia in the general population. It is unknown whether these findings can be generalized to cancer patients, because relevant literature is virtually nonexistent, with few exceptions.

Delirium and terminal restlessness

Prevalence

Delirium is a common disorder in hospitalized, medically ill patients. It is characterized by abrupt onset of disturbances of consciousness, attention, cognition and perception that tend to fluctuate over the day. Delirium is associated with increased morbidity and mortality, and interferes with pain and other symptom management in cancer patients. The elderly, postoperative patients, and cancer and AIDS patients are at greater risk of delirium. Up to 80% of patients with terminal illness develop delirium near death.

Presentation and etiology

The clinical features of delirium are quite numerous and include a variety of neuropsychiatric symptoms, shared by other common psychiatric disorders such as depression, anxiety, dementia and psychosis.

Prodromal symptoms include restlessness, anxiety, sleep disturbance and irritability.

Common clinical features, often rapidly changing and fluctuating, comprise reduced attention; altered arousal; increased or decreased motor activity; disturbance of the sleep–wake cycle; affective symptoms (mood lability, sadness, anger and euphoria); altered perception (misperceptions, illusions and hallucinations); poorly formed delusions, most often paranoid delusions; disorganized thinking and incoherent speech; disorientation in time, space, person and situation; and memory impairment.

Three clinical subtypes of delirium, based on arousal disturbance and psychomotor behavior, have been described: the hyperactive (hyperaroused, hyperalert or agitated) subtype, the hypoactive (hypoaroused, hypoalert or lethargic) subtype, and a mixed subtype with alternating features of the hyper- and hypoactive subtypes.

It has been suggested that the hyperactive form is most often characterized by hallucinations, delusions, agitation and disorientation, whereas the hypoactive form is characterized by confusion and sedation, and is rarely associated with psychotic features. In addition, there is evidence that specific delirium subtypes may have unique pathophysiology and may respond differently to treatment. It is estimated that 75% of all cases of delirium are either of the hypoactive or of the mixed form, whereas the classical hyperactive type of delirium is actually a minority of the cases that occur.

Only a small percentage of delirious patients have a single etiological factor; the condition seems to be essentially multifactorial. Most of those etiologies are putative, and the etiology of 75% of cases remains unknown. For example, a recent study showed that 16% of the sample had one etiological factor, 27% had two and 90% had up to four possible etiologies. The same study failed to correlate the phenomenology of delirium and etiology. In cancer patients, the most frequent etiologies are brain metastases, medication side effects, infections, metabolic disorders due to organ failure and hypoxia.

Diagnosis

The diagnosis relies on the history and the presence of an abruptly altered mental state, with inability to maintain or shift attention and cognitive impairment. It must be remembered that attention deficit fluctuates during the day, and history by family members or chart review is often useful, since patients may have lucid intervals. Moreover, subtle changes in mental status may go unnoticed or be attributed to the stress of cancer. A close watch of mental function and comparison with its prior level help to differentiate delirium from normal stress reactions, adjustment disorder or early dementia. Clinical examination, laboratory data and other investigations assist in establishing etiology. Several assessment instruments have been developed, among them the Memorial Delirium Assessment Scale (MDAS) and the Delirium Rating Scale–Revised (DRS-R) which are mainly utilized for research purposes.

Treatment

Delirium was, by definition, considered to be a transient disorder, most often of brief duration. This statement is no longer valid, since the literature suggests a poorer outcome than previously thought for a large proportion of patients. In a geriatric population, the mortality rate after an episode of delirium reached 30% at 1 year, and 32% of all patients had persistent courses, notably with constant cognitive and functional impairment, irrespective of pre-existing dementia.

The treatment of delirium is a multistep or a multicomponent intervention.

- The underlying causes of delirium have to be identified if possible and treated.
- Several nonpharmacological interventions have proven effective, such as fluid and electrolyte balance, nutrition, and measures to reduce anxiety and disorientation (constant reorientation, correction of hearing and visual impairment, and early mobilization).

- Pharmacological treatment is an important part of the multicomponent intervention.
  - Haloperidol is still considered the reference standard for the treatment of delirious patients. It can be used orally or intravenously with doses that seldom need to exceed 20 mg/day.
  - Olanzapine or risperidone has proven to be a valid alternative for those who have demonstrated intolerance to the extrapyramidal side effects of the classic neuroleptics.
  - A switch to methotrimeprazine is an alternative when agitation is not controlled satisfactorily.
  - In the case of refractory agitation, augmentation of a haloperidol regimen with lorazepam can be useful.
  - Parenteral infusions of midazolam, a short-acting benzodiazepine, or of propofol, a short-acting anesthetic agent, have been used to control agitation related to delirium in the terminally ill. With propofol, the level of sedation is more easily controlled, and recovery is rapid upon decreasing the rate of infusion.
- While there is a consensus on how to treat agitated delirious patients, the management of hypoalert, somnolent patients in terms of pharmacological and nonpharmacological interventions has been studied to a minor extent. However, some evidence has been published on the use of psychostimulants in that population.

Terminal restlessness

Terminal restlessness is common at the end of life. The literature suggests that 25–88% of all dying patients exhibit this condition. It is commonly heralded by agitation, mental anguish and general unease that may appear as thrashing, involuntary muscle twitching or jerks, fidgeting or tossing and turning, or yelling or moaning.

This syndrome is complex, with multiple possible causes, including metabolic disturbance, infection, fear, anxiety, uncontrolled symptoms, drug toxicity, confusion and delirium. Delirium is present most of the time, and terminal restlessness is sometimes considered a particular form of agitated delirium.

It can sometimes be relieved by simple measures such as repositioning the patient or emptying a full bowel or bladder. In many cases, the cause is irreversible, and it is usually impossible to determine all contributory factors. A common management approach is sedation. This is achieved by the administration of benzodiazepines or phenothiazine, either in combination or alone; some protocols advocate the use of ready-made mixtures combining anesthetics, opiates and benzodiazepines.

Further reading

Akechi T Okuyama T, Sugawara Y et al: Major depression, adjustment disorders, and post-traumatic stress disorder in terminally ill cancer patients: associated and predictive factors. J Clin Oncol 2004; 22: 1957–65.

Breitbart W: Diagnosis and management of delirium in the terminally ill. In: Topics in Palliative Care. Oxford: Oxford University Press, 2001.

Cullivan R, Crown J, Walsh N: The use of psychotropic medication in patients referred to a psycho-oncology service. Psychooncology 1998; 7: 301–6.

Mock V: Fatigue management: evidence and guidelines for practice. Cancer 2001; 92 (Suppl): 1699–1707.

Morin CM, Culbert JP, Schwartz SM: Nonpharmacological interventions for insomnia: a meta-analysis of treatment efficacy. Am J Psychiatry 1994; 151: 1172–80.

NCCN Cancer-Related Fatigue Panel: National Comprehensive Cancer Network. Clinical Practice Guidelines in Oncology. Cancer-Related Fatigue Version 2, 2005.

Pezzella G, Moslinger-Gehmayr R, Contu A: Treatment of depression in patients with breast cancer: a comparison between paroxetine and amitriptyline. Breast Cancer Res Treat 2001; 70: 1–10.

Razavi D, Stiefel F: Psychiatric disorders in cancer patients. In: Klastersky J, Schimpff SC, Senn HJ (eds), Supportive Care in Cancer, 2nd edn. New York: Marcel Dekker, 1999.

Sheard T, Maguire P: The effect of psychological interventions on anxiety and depression in cancer patients: results of two meta-analyses. Br J Cancer 1999; 80: 1770–80.

Stiefel F, Berney A, Mazzocato C: Psychopharmacology in supportive care in cancer: a review for the clinician. I. Benzodiazepines. Support Care Cancer 1999; 7: 379–85.

Stiefel F, Stagno D: Management of insomnia in patients with chronic pain conditions. CNS Drugs 2004; 18: 285–96.

15 Cancer pain

M Kloke, S Stevens, M Stahl
Zentrum für Palliativmedizin, Kliniken Essen-Mitte, Germany

Prevalence and etiology

Pain is a complex physiological and emotional experience, and not a simple sensation. It always has social and spiritual components. The experience of chronic pain induces depression, exacerbates anxiety, causes sleep disturbances, contributes to fatigue and general deterioration, and interferes with social activities.

At the time of diagnosis, one-third of cancer patients suffer from pain; in advanced stages, at least two-thirds suffer. Cancer itself causes about 80–90% of pain syndromes; 20–40% are therapy-induced. Only 2–4% of cancer patients suffer from chronic pain unrelated to cancer (e.g. migraine or low back pain). Multiple causes can be present in one patient, one-third of patients suffering from three or more types of pain.

Pain classification and assessment
Types of pain

Pain has physical, psychosocial, emotional and spiritual components. Pain in cancer patients is multidimensional and should be designated as 'total pain' with severe impact on the quality of life and social functioning.

Based on pathophysiology, there are two main types: nociceptive and neuropathic pain, with an increasing number of mixed pain syndromes in advanced cancer (more than 60% of patients suffer from mixed pain). Recent results of tests in animal pain models suggest that pain caused by bone metastasis is a specific entity.

Nociceptive pain (damage to bone, soft tissue or viscera, with physiological pain transmission)

■ Bone or soft-tissue pain: numb, stabbing, exactly localized and frequently movement-induced

- Visceral pain: pressing, deep inside, poorly localized, referred pain and, in the case of bowel obstruction colicky or cramping.

Neuropathic pain (damage to nerve tissues, with altered pain transmission)

- Spontaneous versus provoked
- Continuous versus paroxysmal
- Hot, burning, stabbing or itching.

Neuropathic pain can be accompanied by allodynia, hyperpathy, hyperalgesia, dysesthesia, hypoesthesia, anesthesia and paralysis.

Subtypes of neuropathic pain are as follows:

- peripheral neuropathy
- phantom, central and deafferentation pain
- sympathically maintained pain.

The differentiation between different pain types is based on an exact pain assessment. Since pain is completely subjective, a number of self-assessment tools have been validated (e.g. the Brief Pain Inventory and the McGill Pain Questionnaire), addressing the multidimensional nature of pain and its impact on daily activity and life quality. In addition to anamnesis, nonverbal communication and coping also need to be registered. In patients who are not able to answer questionnaires, pain assessment should adhere to a minimal standardized interview focusing on the following questions:

- Where is the pain (e.g. segmental, nonsegmental; referable to joints, muscles, bone, viscera, peripheral nerve, nerve plexus)?
- What is the pain like (e.g. hot, itchy, numb, throbbing, aching)?
- How strong is the pain (e.g. categorical verbal or numeric rating scale, visual analog scale)?
- What worsens or what ameliorates the pain (e.g. movement, food intake, temperature, bearing, posture)?
- Is the pain stable or are there episodes of recurrent pain (e.g. continuous, circadian rhythm, paroxysmal, breakthrough pain? See Figure 15.1.
- How did the pain develop (e.g. duration, increase or decrease of pain intensity, increase of painful zones or locations)?
- What are the concomitant symptoms (e.g. palpitation, vomiting, nausea, sweating, diarrhea, constipation, dyspnea)?
- How does the pain interfere with activities of daily life (sleep disturbance, restriction in mobility or inability to eat)?

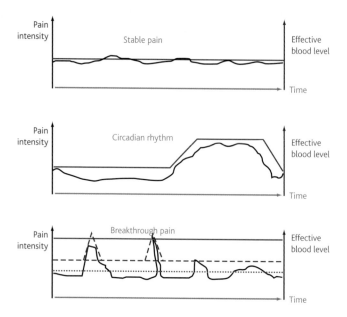

Figure 15.1 Pain modalities

Pain assessment is completed by an accurate physical examination, including a neurological examination. This is necessary before initiating pain therapy and reduces the number of required additional examinations. Before defining the therapeutic concept, additional symptoms in the context of cancer disease have to be taken into account. They can be aggravated (e.g. constipation, nausea, sedation and pruritus) or ameliorated (e.g. dyspnea, cough and diarrhea) by opioids. Sometimes, their adequate palliation has a greater meaning for the patient's well-being than complete pain relief.

Treatment of pain
Multidisciplinary approach

Treatment of pain enforces an interdisciplinary and multiprofessional approach to equilibrate the individual risk–benefit ratio of each therapeutic intervention. This includes disease-modifying therapies (chemotherapy, irradiation and surgery) as well as nonmedical options such as indwelling catheters or stents, physical therapy and psychological support. They are initiated concordantly with the medical pain therapy and adapted according to the patient's needs and treatment options. It is of great importance to develop a 'therapeutic ladder' with clearly defined aims (e.g. first step: sleep will not be interrupted by pain; second: adequate pain control at rest; third: daily activities are not influenced by pain) and to discuss this with the patient. In the course of treatment, routine re-evaluation of efficacy and toxicity is needed.

Principles of medical pain therapy

In 1997, the World Health Organization (WHO) published the second edition of its guidelines on cancer pain therapy. Adhering to these recommendations permits adequate pain control in 80–90% of patients by noninvasive procedures. Additionally, 10% of patients can achieve sufficient pain relief with parenteral, epidural or intrathecal application of analgesics.

Medical pain therapy adheres to certain principles:

- Priority of oral administration: oral administration of drugs has proven to be safe, effective, and easy, supporting the autonomy of patients and keeping them independent of specific medical or technical help. Other routes of administration require specific indications with perhaps one exception – in patients with stable pain, transdermal opioid patches may be equivalent to oral intake. With respect to their bioavailability, which might be altered seriously in cases of organic impairment, the effectiveness of drugs is generally independent of their route of administration. Each route can achieve equipotent blood levels.
- Drugs are administered according to the duration of their activity. This means that medication needs to be taken at fixed time intervals. For dose titration as well as for breakthrough pain, normal-release (NR) or immediate-release (IR) preparations are preferred. After determination of the dose for pain control, sustained-release (SR) formulations are useful. It seems to be advantageous to use the same drug in both situations (Figure 15.2).
- Pain therapy is built up stepwise (the 'analgesic ladder'). Pain therapy is initiated with nonopioids. Weak opioids are added in step II. If pain control remains insufficient, weak opioids are replaced by strong opioids. Nonopioids should be continued in steps II and III (Figure 15.3).
- Depending on the pain modality, coanalgesic drugs can be added at each level.
- Frequent and serious unwanted side effects should be treated prophylactically.

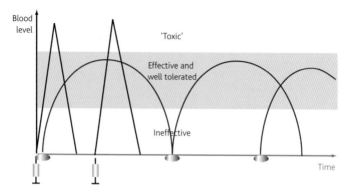

Figure 15.2 *Therapeutic principles: medication should be taken by the mouth and by the clock*

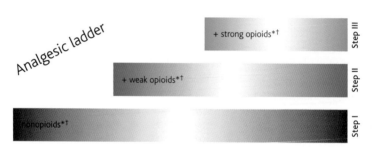

*Coanalgesics recommended according to the pain modality
†Adjuvants as required

Figure 15.3 *WHO analgesic ladder*

- Breakthrough pain requires additional treatment in accordance with pain type.
- In the course of treatment, efficacy, tolerability and safety should be reassessed. This can be done with diaries or ranking scales.

Analgesics
Nonopioids (step I)

Nonopioids are effective in cancer pain therapy. If the individual- and drug-linked risk profiles, contraindications and interactions are considered, these drugs have a tolerable benefit–risk ratio (Table 15.1). Their antipyretic potency needs to be taken into account in the immunosuppressed patient, because this might lead to delayed detection of serious infections.

The effectiveness of paracetamol (acetaminophea) in cancer has never been proved scientifically. In patients with pre-existing (alcoholic) liver disease, hepatotoxicity occurs at daily doses of less than 6 g.

Nonsteroidal anti-inflammatory drugs (NSAIDs) have excellent anti-inflammatory properties. Therefore, they have some advantages in pain caused by bone or periostal metastasis and in inflammatory processes. Their gastrointestinal toxicity increases with the concomitant administration of corticosteroids or aspirin. Patients with a history of ulcers or chronic gastritis should not be treated with NSAIDs. The risk of severe renal toxicity (up to irreversible acute renal failure) increases dramatically in patients with pre existing nephropathy, dehydration, advanced age, hypertension and cardiac insufficiency. NSAIDs interact with the majority of antihypertensive drugs, especially angiotensin-converting enzyme (ACE) inhibitors, oral antidiabetics, diuretics, methotrexate and coumarins. They inhibit platelet aggregation, and caution is recommended in patients with thrombocytopenia or bleeding diathesis. Delirium can occur, especially in elderly patients.

There is only limited evidence of the effectiveness and safety of the new cyclooxygenase-2 (COX-2) inhibitors in cancer pain. They are thought to produce less serious gastrointestinal adverse events. This advantage is lost in patients receiving aspirin or corticosteroids. They have no impact on platelet aggregation, and this might be advantageous in patients with thrombocytopenia. There is an increased risk of thromboembolic complications.

Opioids (steps II and III)

Mode of action

Opioids are safe drugs that are highly effective against pain. The pharmacological effects of opioids are derived from their complex interactions with three main opioid receptors (μ, δ and κ) and subtypes. These receptors are found in the periphery, at presynaptic and postsynaptic sites of the ascending pain transmission system, and in structures that comprise a descending inhibitory system. In spite of the established relationship between site and type of opioid receptor binding and effect (blockade of the μ_1 receptor by naloxonazine abolishes the analgesic effect without influencing either the respiratory depression or the inhibition of gastrointestinal transit), there seem to be individually fixed differences in the opioid response.

Table 15.1 Nonopioid drugs

Substance (mg)	Single dose	Duration of effect (h)	Analgesic potency	Antipyretic	Anti-inflammatory	Spasmolytic
Paracetamol (acetaminophea)	500–1000	4	+	+	–	–
Ibuprofen	400–600* 600–800†	6 8–12	++	++	++	–
Diclofenac	50–100* 100†	6–8 12	+++	++	+++	–
Celecoxib	100–200	24	++	++	++	–

*Normal-release formulation.

†Slow-release formulation.

Several gene polymorphisms have been described, especially for the human μ-opioid receptor gene, resulting in different effects. For example, the A118G polymorphism at the μ-receptor gene significantly reduces the potency of and protects against the toxicity of morphine-6-glucuronide.

There are also substantial differences in the biochemistry of opioids, and these factors interfere with their mode of exerting analgesia. For example, the distribution within the body of the lipophilic methadone and fentanyl differs widely from that of the more hydrophilic morphine and hydromorphone. Metabolic pathways play an important role not only in the bioavailability of opioids (e.g. a reduced first-pass elimination capacity of the liver will increase the bioavailability of oral morphine and hydromorphone) but also in their analgesic potency (e.g. tramadol is less effective in poor metabolizers at the cytochrome P450 isoenzyme CYP2D6, and tilidine needs to be activated within the liver). Impairment of renal function is important in patients treated with morphine due to the accumulation of the active morphine 3- and 6-glucuronides.

All these factors may contribute to the fact that tolerance is incomplete between different opioids and that tachyphylaxis develops discordantly in time and intensity of side effects. This is also reflected by the fact that the prevalence of side effects is closely correlated with the duration of administration of medication. Moreover, these experimental findings agree with the clinical observation that in patients with insufficient pain control or suffering from intolerable side effects, changes of the opioid might dramatically increase analgesia and reduce unwanted side effects.

With respect to the complexity of symptoms in advanced cancer, the entire spectrum of opioid effects should be taken into consideration in order to use opioid side effects (e.g. the antitussive, antidyspnoeic, antidiarrheal effect).

Tachyphylaxis with a specific side effect should be reflected in the recurrence of former symptoms (e.g. nausea with stable dosages for a long period). Further, it is of great importance that opioids lack toxicity directed against a distinct organ or tissue (e.g. any renal, hepatic or bone-marrow toxicity). Therefore, they might be superior to nonopioids in multimorbid or elderly patients. Thus, opioids are the mainstay of cancer pain therapy, and they should not be withheld.

The myth of opioids and its impact on efficacy

There are numerous misunderstandings concerning opioids. These lead to substantial undertreatment of pain, even in patients with advanced cancer, due to severe underdosing or even withholding opioids until the terminal phase. Moreover, the availability of strong opioids is restricted by strict legislation in many European countries. For patients and their relatives, the prescription of opioids is frequently misinterpreted as a major indicator of imminent death, and they fear alterations in perception and emotion and impaired cognitive function. Loss of control over disease progression is also feared, as are addiction or physical dependence and loss of efficacy. To address these issues in an open manner and to discuss fears openly is an essential step in pain therapy. Therefore, physicians must be familiar with opioids and be able to prevent and treat undesirable side effects appropriately.

Opioid effects

Analgesia, tolerance and hyperalgesia

Analgesic potency is fixed by intrinsic activity (IA). The reference substance morphine exhibits an intrinsic activity of 1 and is a complete agonist of the μ receptor. Since naloxone exhibits no IA (IA = 0), it is a complete antagonist of the μ receptor.

Another important characteristic of a substance is its affinity with the μ receptor. Buprenorphine has a low intrinsic activity but a high affinity compared with morphine. This might result in withdrawal symptoms if medication with a full agonist is stopped and replaced by a partial antagonist.

Full μ receptor agonists are thought to lack a ceiling effect: this means that increasing the dose results in better analgesia. The great majority of patients will never stop benefiting from dose escalation if pain is getting worse; for them, tachyphylaxis is without clinical significance.

Opioid tolerance can be defined as the need for dose escalation without increasing nociceptive input, and should be regarded as a normal adaptation process. Receptor changes involved in tolerance comprise different processes:

- Receptor downregulation, which means loss of receptor proteins. This seems not to be the main mechanism in vivo.
- Desensitization based on receptor decoupling, receptor internalization and increased alternative coupling to stimulatory G-proteins has been demonstrated. Since tolerance is incomplete, changing the opioid might be successful in these patients.

For the majority of patients, tolerance is without clinical relevance.

A recently recognized complication of high-dose and prolonged opioid therapy seems to be the phenomenon of hyperalgesia. Although only a few patients develop this painful state, one should consider it if a patient experiences more pain with increasing doses of opioids. This should lead to lowering the dose, adding coanalgesics or searching for alternative methods for pain control.

Nausea and vomiting

Within the first 2 weeks of opioid therapy, 40–60% of patients suffer from nausea and vomiting. This can be caused by different mechanisms: irritation of the dopaminergic D_2 receptor-binding site in the area postrema, delayed gastric emptying and constipation. Therefore, it seems advisable to offer some antiemetics, prophylactically, preferably with D_2 receptor antagonistic activity during this period (e.g. 0.5–1.5 mg haloperidol/day or 20–30 mg metoclopramide/day).

If the irritation of the chemoreceptor trigger zone activates the vomiting center, antihistaminergic, antimuscarinic or anticholinergic drugs might be added, but at the cost of losing the prokinetic action of metoclopramide or domperidone (e.g. dimenhydrinate, cyclizine, scopolamine, butylscopolamine).

If nausea recurs while the patient is on a stable opioid dose, other causes need to be ruled out (e.g. hypercalcemia, cerebral metastasis, bowel obstruction, metabolic disorders with accumulation of opioid metabolites or increased bioavailability due to decreased metabolism).

Sedation/delirium

Sedation is a regular reaction of the body when opioid therapy is started. It is more pronounced in elderly and cachectic patients, and is intensified by comedication with other centrally acting drugs (e.g. benzodiazepines, antidepressants, neuroleptics and antihypertensive drugs). In the majority of patients, sedation will be reduced or even disappear in the course of treatment. If it persists or is complicated by delirium or confusion, lowering the dose or changing the opioid needs to be considered. It is advisable to inform the patient and relatives about the tachyphylaxis of this frightening symptom in order to enhance compliance.

The recurrence of sedation and confusion in patients on stable doses must initiate an evaluation of other causes.

The patient must be instructed about the possibly reduced ability to drive and to work with dangerous machines. A small number of patients suffer from ongoing sedation. Although this should be considered to be multicausal in the majority (e.g. concomitant fatigue, cachexia, muscle weakness and general deterioration), sometimes the addition of amphetamines or modafinil is helpful for a limited period.

Constipation

Constipation is the most common and persistent side effect of opioids. It causes nausea, vomiting, and loss of appetite and weight; it impairs general well-being and activity; and it can be dangerous when it leads to bowel obstruction. Constipation is mediated by the central nervous system (brain and spinal cord) as well as by the intestinal nervous system (opioid receptors within the plexus myentericus). The increased tone of the intestinal smooth muscles, the loss of the large migrating complexes, and the increased tone of the intestinal sphincters delay the progress of intestinal contents. This prolonged transit phase increases reabsorption of water. Moreover, the binding of opioids reduces intestinal secretion, thus contributing to hard stools.

The increased use of transdermal patches initiated a discussion of whether constipation is related to drug, application mode or dosage. Today, there is some evidence that constipation might be less severe with transdermal fentanyl or buprenorphine patches than with oral opioids.

Constipation increases rather than decreases in the course of treatment. Therefore its prophylactic treatment is obligatory regardless of poor patient compliance. A stepwise approach can be used (Figure 15.4).

Respiratory depression

The respiratory depressant potency of opioids is correlated with their intrinsic activity at the μ receptor and is characterized by rapid tachyphylaxis. Respiratory depression hardly ever occurs if the dose has been titrated correctly and with oral therapy. It should not be confused with dyspnea (the subjective sensation of difficult breathing).

For this dangerous side effect to occur, a massive overdosing, mostly in combination with other centrally acting drugs, especially benzodiazepines, is needed. This can mostly be related to the fact that the breathing center within the formatio reticularis is hyperactivated by pain and is reduced to normal in a pain-free status.

If the antidyspneic potency of opioids is the focus of therapy, a dose escalation of at least 30% is required compared with the analgesic dosages in order to achieve an effect.

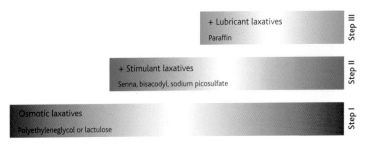

Combination of drugs is advisable in order to reduce side effects.
Rectal laxatives can be used in addition.

Figure 15.4 Laxative ladder for opioid-induced constipation

In daily clinical practice, counting the frequency of breathing can be used to decide whether there is a severe overdosing of opioids (fewer than 10 breaths per minute). In a conscious patient, a command to breathe may be helpful.

Naloxone needs to be used cautiously. The one exception to the rule is in patients with (pre)terminal renal insufficiency, in whom the active metabolite morphine 6-glucuronide might accumulate and exert a profound respiratory depression. In patients with renal failure, the use of opioids without active metabolites and/or only partial excretion by the kidneys seems to be advisable.

Antitussive effect

Suppression of the protective cough reflex is maximal at dosages below those required for analgesia. It is not correlated with μ receptor binding and is stronger with codeine, hydrocodeine, dihydrocodeine and oxycodone than with morphine, hydromorphone and fentanyl at equianalgesic dosages. Tachyphylaxis quickly develops.

Urinary retention

Urinary retention occurs predominantly in patients with pre-existing disorders, such as neurogenic dysuria or benign prostatic hypertrophy. This can be treated medically with carbachol (10–40 mg/day) or phenoxybenzamine (10–40 mg/day). Sometimes, a urinary catheter is necessary. Tachyphylaxis is not relevant.

Pruritus

Opioids may cause pruritus, especially within the perioral zone, without any skin reaction. This side effect is more frequent in spinal opioid therapy and usually disappears gradually. Patients must be instructed that this phenomenon is different from allergy.

Physical and psychological dependence

There can be no doubt of the potency of opioids to induce *habituation dependence*. Addicts crave the drug in order to experience its psychotropic effects regardless of the detrimental effects of its use. Since the driving power of this behavior is euphoria, which is nearly never observed in patients receiving opioids for analgesic purposes, psychological dependence is not induced by the proper use of opioids. However, a history of substance abuse has proved to be a poor prognostic factor for adequate pain control.

Physical dependence is characterized by withdrawal symptoms when the drug is stopped suddenly. If the nociceptive input is reduced and the patient needs smaller dosages or even does not need more opioids, dose reduction by about 10% per day will be possible without causing withdrawal symptoms. It is important to be aware of the early signs of withdrawal (jawing, diarrhea, sweating and restlessness), since the patient may have serious problems without treatment. Careful titration with normal-release opioid formulations is the appropriate way to deal with those problems in palliative medicine.

Weak opioids (step II)

Weak and strong opioids share the same pattern of side effects. Their effectiveness in cancer pain has been proven. Their analgesic potency is estimated to be one-tenth or one-fifth that of oral morphine. The drugs in this group have a ceiling effect, which means that from a clinical point of view their maximum achievable analgesic effect is limited. They can be combined with nonopioids.

Codeine

About 5–10% of Caucasians are poor CYP2D6 metabolizers. This means that they will not experience adequate pain control with codeine. Moreover, severe interactions are possible with chlorpromazine, haloperidol, levomepromazine metoclopramide and tricyclic antidepressants. In the case of compromised liver function, the efficacy of codeine is reduced. Codeine is frequently used in compound analgesics. A single dose (SD) is 30–40 mg and the duration of effect (DE) is 4 hours.

Dihydrocodeine

Twice as potent as codeine, dihydrocodeine is metabolized in the liver and has the same interaction profile as codeine. Like codeine, it has excellent antitussive and antidiarrheal efficacy. For a normal-release (NR) formulation, SD is 10–20 mg and DE is 4 hours; for a sustained-release (SR) formulation, SD is 60 mg and DE is 12 hours.

Tramadol

This is a weak μ-opioid agonist with additional noradrenergic and serotoninergic effects. Since it is metabolized in the liver and excreted renally, dose adaptation is required in the case of renal insufficiency. Combination with serotonin reuptake inhibitors (e.g. paroxetine) can induce a serotoninergic syndrome. For an NR formulation, SD is 50–100 mg and DE is 4–6 hours; for an SR formulation, SD is 100–200 mg and DE is 12 hours. An intravenous application is also available, with a bioavailability of 100%.

The tolerability of the formulations seems to be superior to that of the NR formulations, with less nausea and orthostatic complaints.

Tildine/naloxone

In this compound drug, tildine is activated by the liver and naloxone is inactivated by the liver. Since the first-pass elimination capacity is highly individual, efficacy varies widely. For an NR formulation, SD is 50–100 mg and DE is 4–6 hours; for an SR formulation, SD is 100–200 mg and DE is 12 hours.

Pentazocine and pethidine (meperidine)

Pentazocine can produce psychotomimetic effects, including hallucinations, while pethidine (meperidine) can provoke central hyperexcitation, including convulsions. Neither drug can now be recommended for cancer patients.

Strong opioids (step III)

Step III opioids can be divided into two groups: μ receptor agonists (morphine, hydromorphone, oxycodone, L-methadone and fentanyl) and partial antagonists such as buprenorphine.

Buprenorphine and perhaps oxycodone have a ceiling effect, limiting, from the clinical point of view, dose escalation. Although the analgesic potency of these substances has been calculated from data obtained by single-dose experiments, there is a wide range of real equianalgesic doses between individuals.

Morphine remains the reference drug due to the enormous clinical experience and the availability of morphine preparations for each route of administration. At present, little is known about specific circumstances favoring one opioid over another and selection if generally made by personal choice. This has to be taken into account when an opioid rotation is performed.

Morphine

Morphine is still the strong opioid of choice (perhaps more by history than by rationale). It binds to all types of opioid receptors. The main metabolic pathway of morphine is glucuronidation within the liver leading to two active metabolites: morphine 6-glucuronide (up to 20 times more potent at the μ receptor than morphine) and 3-glucuronide (acting as a central excitatory substance). Since these are excreted together with morphine by the kidneys, great care should be taken in patients with renal impairment, and morphine should be avoided in the case of terminal renal insufficiency. Interactions with other drugs, however, are without relevance. The oral bioavailability is 30% in repeated doses, and this can increase dramatically in the case of liver failure.

Morphine is available as NR and SR formulations for oral and rectal application, and it can be used subcutaneously and intraveneously, as well as epidurally or intrathecally. It is important to note that analgesia will not occur before at least 30 minutes after oral intake of the NR preparation, and 20 minutes after intravenous application, with maximum effect after 1 hour. SR morphine will not reach its complete effectiveness before 60 minutes. SR tablets should not be broken. SR capsules can be opened without loss of effect. For patients with difficulty in swallowing, a SR liquid preparation is available (Table 15.2).

Hydromorphone

Hydromorphone is similar to morphine and is metabolized within the liver with an insignificant portion of 3-glucuronide. It is eliminated by the kidneys and requires dose adaptation in renal impairment. Relevant pharmacological interactions with other substances are not known. The oral bioavailability is 40% and increases with liver failure.

Table 15.2 Morphine: preparations and indications

Application mode	Single dose	Duration of effect	Indications	Preparations
Oral immediate release	From 5 mg	4 hours	Dose titration Breakthrough pain	Tablets, drops syrup
Rectal immediate release	From 5 mg	4 hours	Breakthrough pain Dose titration Oral intake impossible	Suppositories
Oral sustained release	From 10 mg	8–12 hours	Basic medication	Tablets, capsules, liquids
Intravenous subcutaneous	From 2 mg	4 hours	Oral intake impossible, rapid dose titration required	Concentrations up to 20 mg/ml available
Epidural/ intrathecal	Individual dose titration required	Late respiratory depression possible	Inadequate pain control and intolerable side effects with the (par)enteral route	Different methods used

It can be given subcutaneously, intravenously and orally.

For an NR formulation, SD is from 1.3 mg and DE is 4 hours per capsule; for an SR formulation, SD is from 4 mg and DE is 12 hours. Its equianalgesic potency compared with morphine is 5–7.5. Since there are no relevant active metabolites, it may be safer and better tolerated in multimorbid and elderly patients.

Fentanyl

Fentanyl is a selective μ-receptor agonist and is highly lipophilic. It can therefore be administered by the transdermal or transmucosal route. It is metabolized by the liver to inactive products. It is highly protein-bound (85%), possibly interacting with other drugs. The indication for the patch is restricted to stable pain conditions without any circadian rhythm. It takes 12–24 hours to reach therapeutic blood levels, and approximately 72 hours to reach steady state. Up to 25% of patients need a change of the patch every 48 hours instead of 72 hours. Absorption might increase up to 30% in fever and decrease during profound sweating. It is important to adhere strictly to the application prescriptions for safety. A 25 μg/h releasing patch is equivalent to a daily dose of 0.6 mg intravenous fentanyl or 60 mg oral morphine. The smallest patch delivers 12.5 μg/hour.

For breakthrough pain, an oral transmucosal fentanyl (OTF) lozenge has been developed. However, the bioavailability of OTF varies widely not only between individuals but also intraindividually. Therefore, it is recommended always to start with a 200 μg lozenge. Careful adherence to the application prescription is needed to obtain its full effectiveness.

Methadone

Methadone is a racemate isomer consisting of the R and the inactive S isomer. In some European countries, a pure preparation of the S form is used for analgesia and the racemate for substitution. It acts as an agonist at the μ and δ receptors and as an antagonist at the N-methyl-D-aspartate (NMDA) receptor. Another nonopioid analgesic receptor activity is the prevention of monamine reuptake in the periaquaductal gray area.

There is some clinical evidence that if an opioid change is recommended in complicated neuropathic pain, methadone might have some superiority. Nevertheless, this substance needs to be used with caution due to its highly individualized pharmacokinetics and pharmacodynamics. Steady state is reached within 20–200 hours. Methadone is metabolized in the liver predom-

Table 15.3 *Interactions of methadone with other drugs*

Drugs whose serum levels are increased by methadone	Desimipramine, zidovudine
Drugs reducing methadone clearance	Fluconazole, fluoxetine, fluvoxamine, ketoconazole
Drugs increasing methadone clearance	Carbamazepine, chronic alcohol abuse, fusidic acid, phenytoin, resperidone, rifampicin, ritonavir
Drugs leading to synergistic toxicity	Benzodiazepines
Drugs providing synergistic analgesia	Dronabinol, ibuprofen

inantly by CYP1A2, CPY3A and CPY2B6, resulting in common and severe interactions with frequently used substances (Table 15.3).

Methadone can be used in renal impairment because there are no active metabolites. Sixty percent of methadone is excreted by nonrenal routes (e.g. stools). Low urinary pH levels increase renal clearance threefold. The oral bioavailability is about 80%, with a poor subcutaneous tolerability (intravenous administration is possible without problems). For a NR formulation SD is from 2.5 mg orally or 2 mg intravenously. In contrast to substitution therapy, the analgesic DE is 8–12 hours, requiring twice daily application. Equipotency of doses when changing to methadone is correlated with the duration and the dosages of pretreatment with the previous opioid. Various methods for changing to methadone are used in Europe (Tables 15.4a and b).

Oxycodone

Oxycodone is metabolized in the liver to active oxymorphone. Its oral bioavailability is about 60%, and it is eliminated by the kidneys. Relevant interaction might occur with substances using the CYP2D6 metabolic pathway. Oxycodone binds at the μ and κ receptors. Since its receptor affinity is still not clear, it is used as a step II opioid with a ceiling dose.

It is available as NR tablets and syrup (SD from 5 mg, DE 4 hours) and an SR preparation (SD from 10 mg, DE 12 hours). Its antitussive efficacy seems to be higher, and its antidyspneic potency lower than those of morphine at equianalgesic doses. There is some evidence that it might be useful in patients suffering especially from excitatory opioid side effects. Oxycodone is approximately 1.2–2 times more potent than oral morphine.

Table 15.4a Method for changing to methadone in UK

Step	Procedure
I	Stop morphine
II For daily dose of oral morphine <300 mg	Give a fixed dose of methadone at one-tenth of the daily dose of oral morphine
II For daily dose of oral morphine >300 mg	Give a fixed dose of methadone of 30 mg
III	The fixed dose is taken as needed, but not more frequently than every 3 hours
IV	On day 6, add the total dose of methadone administered in the last 48 hours and give at 12-hour intervals
V For dose adjustment or breakthrough pain	10–15% of daily methadone dose

Table 15.4b Method for changing to methadone in Italy

Step	Procedure
I	Stop morphine
II	Give methadone at fixed intervals every 8 hours
III For daily dose of oral morphine < 90 mg	Methadone:morphine = 1/4
III For daily dose of oral morphine 90–300 mg	Methadone:morphine = 1/8
III For daily dose or oral morphine > 300 mg	Methadone:morphine = 1/12
IV for breakthrough pain	10% of daily methadone dose

Buprenorphine

Buprenorphine is a partial agonist with a ceiling dose of approximately 4 mg/day. It should not be combined with μ agonistic drugs. It is metabolized in the liver. Seventy percent of the drug is eliminated in stools. It is perhaps less spasmogenic at the intestinal sphincters than μ agonists. Since buprenorphine is very lipophilic, it is suitable for transdermal and sublingual use. The indication for the transdermal patch is restricted to stable pain. The patches cover a large area, and therefore only moderate to severe cancer pain can be treated. Local skin reactions must lead to removal of the patch.

SD is from 0.2 mg sublingually and 0.15 mg intravenously; DE is 6–8 hours. Patches reach a stable state after 48–72 hours, with a change every 72 hours. In changing from the transdermal to the sublingual route, a factor of 1.5 may be used. Buprenorphine is thought to be 20–30 times more potent than morphine.

Changing opioids (opioid rotation)

Opioids are highly effective, well-tolerated and low-toxicity drugs. Nevertheless, a substantial number of patients do not achieve sufficient pain control, or they experience intolerable side effects. From clinical experience, it is known that in 60% of these patients, changing the opioid will result in optimized analgesia and abolish intolerable side effects. A multitude of possible explanations have been put forward either from experimental research or animal studies:

- genetic variability of opioid receptors and transport mechanisms
- substance-linked interference with different neuromodulatory systems
- differences in pharmacogenetics and pharmacodynamics
- influences of the cancer cells themselves expressing opioid receptors.

It is recommended that one calculate the equianalgesic dose from the results of single-dose experiments and then reduce it by about 30% (Table 15.5). These doses need to be adapted by titration with NR preparations of the same drug if available. For changing to methadone, a separate dose-finding scheme is required (Tables 15.4a, b).

Changing the route of administration

Transdermal patches

The indication for transdermal patches is restricted to patients with stable pain. Nevertheless, patient compliance and user comfort have led to the wide acceptance of this route of administration. Changing from oral medication is performed by applying the patch concomitantly with the last intake of an SR preparation. Switching to oral medication requires careful titration with NR preparations after removal of the patch, due to its long duration of action. It is unnecessary to start transdermal systems in the terminal phase, since it will take too long to reach therapeutic levels, absorption remains uncertain in altered perfusion, and titration is not possible.

Table 15.5 *Equianalgesic doses of strong opioids*

First-line opioid	Conversion factor	New opioid
Oral morphine	0.13–2	Oral hydromorphone
	0.5	Oral oxycodone
	See Tables 15.4a, b	Oral methadone
	1/ 60	Intravenous fentanyl*
	0.03	Sublingual buprenorphine†
Oral hydromorphone	5-7.50	Oral morphine
Oral oxycodone	2	Oral morphine
Oral methadone	See Tables 15.4a, b: reverse procedure	Oral morphine
Intravenous fentanyl*	60	Oral morphine
Sublingual buprenorphine†	20–30	Oral morphine

* 0.6 mg/d i.v. is equivalent to a patch delivering 25 µg fentanyl/h.

†0.8 mg/d s.l. is equivalent to a patch delivering 35 µg buprenorphine/h.

Parenteral analgesia (intravenous/subcutaneous)

Every fifth patient needs parenteral analgesia, mostly in the terminal phase. The reason for discontinuing oral administration may be the inability to swallow, neurological deficits of the cranial nerves, persistent vomiting, bowel obstruction, impaired cognition, coma or even the need for rapid dose titration.

Dose conversion is performed according to the specific bioavailability of a drug. Usually, changing the application mode while maintaining the drug is without problems except in patients with reduced first-pass elimination capacity or genetic variants.

If permanent intravenous access is present (a subcutaneous portal system or central venous catheter), it can be used for therapy even in outpatients.

An alternative route is a subcutaneous catheter. For this purpose, a small needle is inserted subcutaneously and then fixed with a transparent dressing. It can be left in place for several days.

Pyoderma, anasarca and severe bleeding diathesis are contraindications for subcutaneous administration.

The majority of substances used for pain or symptom control can be given subcutaneously, although this is not advised by the manufacturers. Moreover, a multitude of useful mixtures can be considered as stable for several days (Table 15.6).

Drugs can be either administered as boluses at fixed intervals according to their DE with an appropriate rescue medication, or given continuously by a syringe driver or a small transportable pump (driven by battery or mechanically). The subcutaneous route is very helpful under certain conditions and can be managed even by nonprofessional caregivers.

Use of naloxone

Naloxone acts as an antagonist at the opioid receptor, thus neutralizing the effects of other opioid drugs and endogenous opioids. The first-pass elimination capacity of the liver for oral naloxone varies widely. DE is about 70 minutes. Naloxone is a specific antidote in opioid overdosing, especially in respiratory depression. The required dosage needs to be titrated against effect while trying to avoid withdrawal symptoms as well as recurrent pain. Overdosing of naloxone can cause a fluid lung, and rapid infusion leads to extensive catecholamine secretion with severe arrhythmia.

If the patient is overdosed with NR opioids, 1 ml of diluted naloxone (0.4 mg in 10 ml 0.9% NaCl) is given subcutaneously or intravenously every 3 minutes until the desired effect is observed. This procedure can be repeated if necessary after 1 hour.

Table 15.6 Stability of mixtures for parenteral application

Morphine with	Duration of stability	Indications (except pain)
Haloperidol*	14 days	Sedation, antiemesis, hallucinations
Levomepromazine*	24 hours	Sedation, antiemesis
Chlorpromazine*	>15 min	Sedation, antiemesis, pruritus
Butylscopolamine	24 hours	Spasm of smooth muscles, colic
Midazolam*	4 hours	Sedation, terminal delirium, agitation
Hydrocortison*	>4 hours	Edema, inflammation
Glucose (pH<7)*	24 hours	Hypoglycemia

*Mixtures are suitable for subcutaneous application.

In patients with SR opioids or patches, 2 mg naloxone should be diluted in 500 ml with 0.9% NaCl. The infusion rate is correlated with the effect. This has to be maintained up to 8–24 hours. After recovery, dose titration with NR preparations seems to be advisable.

Coanalgesic or adjuvant drugs

Definition of coanalgesic or adjuvant drugs

Coanalgesic or adjuvant drugs can be defined as substances that are effective in distinct pain conditions without exerting a proper antinociceptive effect. They act via different mechanisms, most of which remains unclear. Coanalgesics can be given at each step of the analgesic ladder. With regard to the additional side effects and interactions that they might produce, their use needs thorough consideration. However, especially in neuropathic pain, they seem to have a place. Their efficacy has been proven in studies dealing with noncancer pain patients, but there is a lack of sufficient evidence of their role in cancer pain.

Coanalgesics in neuropathic pain, including phantom limb and deafferentation pain

Sixty percent of cancer pain syndromes are at least partially caused by damage to neuronal tissue. From the clinical perspective, it is reasonable to differentiate between continuous dysesthetic and paroxsymal neuropathic pain, although no strict correlation can be found between mechanism of nerve injury and pain modality. Neuropathic pain is not opioid-resistant; however, the majority of neuropathic pain conditions – especially the paroxysmal type – are less responsive and require either higher dosing of opioids, with possibly increasing side effects, or the addition of coanalgesics.

Antidepressants

If the pain is dysesthetic and constant and burning, tricylic antidepressants (TCAs) have proven to be effective at doses far below those used for treating depression. The more sedating amitriptyline or doxepine is given at bedtime, starting with 10 or 25 mg and not exceeding 75–100 mg/day. The activating clomipramine should be administered in the morning. It is important to increase the doses slowly, especially in elderly and dehydrated patients. Orthostatic hypotension often causes falls especially in fragile and cachectic patients. Cardiac arrhythmia and severe cardiac insufficiency are contraindications, as are glaucoma or severe liver insufficiency. The seizure potential is increased in patients with pre-existing epilepsy.

Selective serotonin reuptake inhibitors (SSRIs) are thought to exert coanalgesic activity; the function of norepinephrine reuptake inhibitors remains unclear; they may have some effect in selected patients.

Antiepileptic drugs

The newer antiepileptic drugs (AEDs) gabapentin and pregabalin have proven efficacy in both continuous and lancinating neuropathic pain. Since their absorption from the intestines is not proportional to administered doses, there is a wide range of recommended and used dosages: for gabapentin, SD is 200–1200 mg and DE is 8 hours; for pregabalin, SD is 75–150 mg and DE 12 is hours.

They are not metabolized and are eliminated by the kidneys. Dose reduction is strongly recommended in the case of renal insufficiency, but they can be used even in patients on hemodialysis, according to the manufacturers. They have no relevant interactions or contraindications. Side effects are drowsiness, sedation, weight gain, edema and, very rarely confusion.

Carbamazepine is the AED traditionally used in neuralgic pain states. It is important to increase the dose slowly and to titrate it with respect to effectiveness and toxicity (SD 200–300 mg, DE 8–12 hours). Carbamazepine is contraindicated in the case of severe hepatic and cardiac insufficiency or bone marrow depression. Routine assessment of blood cytology, as well as of liver enzymes, is required. Drowsiness, dizziness, skin reactions, nausea, sedation, elevated liver enzymes and thrombocytopenia/leukopenia are frequent side effects. In general, 600–900 mg/day is prescribed.

Due to their side effects and toxicity, the AEDs clonazepam and valproic acid are used only as third-line coanalgesics. Nevertheless, they are worthwhile in patients requiring parenteral therapy, since they are available for both oral and parenteral administration, in contrast to carbamazepine and pregabalin and gabapentin, which are available only for oral intake. Coanalgesic properties have been reported for phenytoin, lamotrigine and oxcarbazepine.

All AEDs are used in doses similiar to those of anticonvulsive treatment with slowly increasing doses. With all AEDs, it is important to monitor effects and side effects carefully to detect severe toxicity at an early state.

Corticosteroids

Corticosteroids are effective in neuropathic pain by reducing the concomitant edema.

NMDA receptor antagonists

The NMDA receptor antagonists ketamine and esketamine should be reserved for complicated pain syndromes. In doses up to 50 and 25 mg respectively per day, nightmares rarely occur. If higher doses are needed, a benzodiazepine is required to prevent nightmares. Hypersecretion of the tracheobronchial system is sometimes a problem.

Phantom limb pain

The incidence of phantom limb pain is correlated with the duration and intensity of pre-existing and postoperative pain. Therefore, optimized analgesic therapy should be delivered before, during and after amputation. Pre-emptive analgesia with epidurally administered local anesthetics is controversial. It is hypothesized that spinally administered local anesthetics prevent deafferentation pain by an α-sympathetic block. The only drug with proven efficacy in phantom limb pain is calcitonin. However, there is uncertainty about the dosage and duration of medication. It remains unclear whether nasal, subcutaneous and intravenous application are equipotent. TCAs and AEDs have only moderate efficacy in phantom limb pain. In persistent stump or deafferentation pain, opioids might be effective, especially if the history of pain is relatively short.

Coanalgesics in bone pain

Pain due to bone metastasis or primary bone cancer often requires high opioid doses and is complicated by movement-induced breakthrough pain. Corticosteroids and NSAIDs act via their anti-inflammatory action. Third- and fourth-generation bisphosphonates provide a proper analgesic effect by modulating the immune mediator response to osteolysis. This effect can be observed in selected patients within a few days and precedes the analgesic effect due to recalcification, which will take several months. Breakthrough pain can be palliated with NR morphine, hydromorphone or oral transmucosal fentanyl at adequate doses (SD is about one-sixth of the routine daily dose). For this type of pain, nonmedical options such as irradiation, application of radioisotopes, corsets and other orthetics are of special value.

Coanalgesics in muscle pain

It is important to distinguish between two types of painful muscle states, since they require completely different medical and nonmedical treatment:

- painful muscle tension generated by the muscles themselves
- muscle spasm deriving from damage to neuronal tissue.

Fear, anxiety, malposition due to bone metastasis, abnormal body position and pain itself result in painful muscle tension. Primarily, these painful states should be approached by nonmedical techniques. If these fail or cannot be executed, benzodiazepines are effective, since they act as muscle relaxants. Many patients welcome their additional anxiolytic potency, although their sedative effect is highly problematic, especially in patients receiving opioids. Since they quickly cause physical habituation, the duration of benzodiazepine intake should be limited if possible.

Painful muscle spasm results from injuries to the spinal cord, cerebral affects or infiltration of the neuronal plexus. Moreover, painful myoclonus is a well-known side effect of opioids, especially in high doses or in cases of renal impairment. Since opioids increase the muscle tone, pain due to muscle spasm can even be aggravated by opioids. Therefore, myotonolytics are needed in this type of pain.

Baclofen is the drug usually used, at a daily dose of 10–60 mg (oral application only). It lowers the threshold for seizures. Alternative drugs are tizanidine, tolpiserone and dantrolene. In the case of inadequate palliation or side effects, changing the myotonolytic substance might be helpful because these substances have different action mechanisms. All of these drugs need to be titrated individually and slowly increased in dose. Baclofen is the drug of choice in hiccup (spasm of the diaphragm; see Chapter 17).

Coanalgesics in colic

Colic due to compression or obstruction of the intestines, the bilary or pancreatic ducts, or the ureters is usually accompanied by vegetative symptoms such as nausea, vomiting, tachycardia or sweating. Therefore oral intake of analgesics is often limited.

Scopolamine and N-butylscopolamine are effective. They have two disadvantages: effective blood levels require the transdermal or parenteral route, and they have serious side effects such as lowering the threshold for seizures and tachycardia.

Corticosteroids might contribute to analgesia by their antiedematous effect.

Complicated pain syndromes
Negative predictors for efficacy

Despite the success rate in cancer pain treatment by the WHO guidelines, there remain a number of patients who fail to obtain adequate pain control with tolerable side effects, or in whom pain control requires enormous efforts.

Bruera and his colleagues were the first to describe five risk factors for inadequate pain control: neuropathic pain, breakthrough pain, history of substance abuse and addiction, need for a rapid escalation of opioid dose not correlated with an increase in the nociceptive input, and unresolved psychosocial problems. Knowledge of these negative predictors is essential to develop a therapeutic concept with realistic aims together with the patient and to face ongoing problems.

Opioid-resistant pain

A few years ago, neuropathic pain was considered to be opioid-resistant. If we compare the numbers needed to treat (NNT) for achieving 50% pain reduction in peripheral neuropathy or trigeminal neuropathy, there is no important difference between TCAs or AEDs and opioids, suggesting that this type of pain is principally opioid-responsive but perhaps at higher doses than those in nociceptive pain.

When cancer patients report pain, they give notice of an unpleasant experience resulting from a complex biopsychosocial process. Spiritual pain cannot be treated with opioids or psychotropic drugs. The same is true of pain due to mourning or imminent departure from life. These opioid-resistant pain states need to be distinguished from hyperalgesic states and opioid tolerance.

Anesthetic methods for pain control
Spinal analgesia (epidural/subarachnoidal)

About 1–2% of patients need spinal analgesia. Drugs can be applied in either the epidural or the subarachnoidal space. These procedures have a distinct indication because complications are frequent and severe. The most common technical problems are dislocation, local fibrosis, and occlusion or fracture of the catheter. More serious complications are infections with sepsis, epidural abscess, meningitis and encephalitis.

For subarachnoidal therapy, an implantable pump system should be used, while for epidural therapy, medication can be given as single boluses, although it is safer and better tolerated when given by continuous application using external pumps. For permanent use, it is recommended that the catheter be externalized by tunneling it subcutaneously away from the spine. If the therapy is scheduled for several weeks, a port system needs to be inserted.

There is little evidence that pain resistant to systemic opioids can be palliated with spinal opioids alone. While nausea, emesis and constipation, as well as dizziness and sedation, seem to be less severe, pruritus and urinary retention are more frequent with spinal opioids. The improved tolerability of spinal opioids can be referred mostly to the dose-reducing effect of this route of administration. The more lipophilic substances such as sufentanil and fentanyl reach their maximal effect within the segments nearest to the tip of the catheter. The hydrophilic morphine and hydromorphone are distributed through the spinal venous plexus and the cerebrospinal fluid, and reach the formatio reticularis after 8–12 hours. They can cause delayed respiratory depression. In switching from systemic to spinal opioids, individual dose titration is required.

In complicated pain syndromes, the addition of local anesthetics, such as bupivacaine or ropivacaine epidurally, is helpful. Their effectiveness depends on the volume and the concentration of the applied drug. It is important to balance analgesic and motor-paralyzing effects. The mechanism of the analgesic effect of spinal clonidine is not yet known. There is clinical evidence of its coanalgesic properties in neuropathic and poorly opioid-responsive pain syndromes.

Neurolysis

Role of neurolysis

The importance of neurolysis in cancer pain treatment has diminished over the last decade with improved medical options. Neurolysis is applicable only in patients with limited life expectancy because deafferentiation pain might be worse than the original pain. The personal experience that is essential to execute these procedures with an acceptable risk–benefit ratio, is restricted to a minority of physicians. Therefore, only a few interventions are relevant in cancer patients.

Each neurolysis procedure requires a normal coagulation status and should be executed only under resuscitation conditions. A trial block must have been successful with acceptable side effects before definite neurolysis.

Celiac plexus block

The celiac plexus is responsible for transmission of nociceptive information from nearly the entire abdomen except the descending colon and the pelvis. Neurolysis has been shown to be effective in pain due to pancreatic cancer or metastases in other upper abdominal viscera. Somatic pain deriving from invasion of the abdominal wall or other somatic structures cannot be palliated by this method. For the experienced physician, the block is time-effective and relatively safe.

Complications are orthostatic hypotension, diarrhea, abdominal aortic dissection, paraplegia and motor paralysis, with an incidence of severe adverse events of 1–3%. The duration of the analgesic effect is from 2 weeks up to 4 months. It can be repeated.

Lysis of the sympathetic chain

Sympathetically maintained pain (e.g. subtypes of neuropathic pain with infiltration of the pelvic structures), pain due to arterial occlusive disease or phantom limb pain sometimes responds to blocks or lysis of the stellate ganglion and the lumbar or the thoracic sympathetic chain.

Other neurolytic procedures

The saddle block is a modified spinal technique of injecting phenol into the cerebrospinal fluid in the lumbar area. This technique is indicated in pain within the perianal area and the perineum. There is a considerable risk of permanent sphincter dysfunction afterward (up to 10%). Therefore, it should be reserved for patients with enterostoma and urostoma.

Rib metastases can cause severe mixed pain syndromes. Blockade or neurolysis of the intercostal nerves (two segments are needed for one rib) provides excellent analgesia for a certain period. A relevant complication of this method is the occurrence of deafferentation pain resistant to treatment.

Nonpharmacological pain interventions
Medical techniques

There are a large number of other methods of pain palliation. Among them, nerve-stimulating procedures, such as acupuncture or transdermal electrostimulation, might be tried under certain circumstances.

Massage, cold/warm packs and physical therapy are effective in cancer patients with pain from skeletal muscles or malposition within the skeletal system. Lymphatic drainage reduces pain in lymphedema.

Adequate care of wounds and pressure sores contributes to pain control. Since local anesthetics exert local toxicity and promote perhaps enlargement of wounds, their use should be limited. Debate continues on whether topically applied opioids act via binding to local opioid receptors or systemically after absorption by the subcutaneous space.

For the palliation of movement-induced pain, the use of corsets and other orthetics, as well as optimized prosthetics, is strongly recommended, since the dosages of opioids needed for adequate control of this type of breakthrough pain are beyond tolerability and induce sedation.

Psychological and spiritual interventions

In accordance with the burden of suffering, the evaluation of unresolved psychological conflicts should be done by either an experienced physician or a psychotherapist. Art, music and speech therapies are helpful if the patient has enough strength to adhere to them, and if they are available. Empathy and encouraging the family and friends to give support can be a worthwhile contribution to pain palliation.

Diagnosing spiritual pain and responding to it adequately remain difficult and require a holistic approach to the patient in pain. Guilt, fear of the imminence of death, mourning, and questioning the sense of suffering and life can be reasons for unresolved pain. These patients are greatly in need of experienced spiritual help.

Conclusion

Pain is one of the most burdensome and common symptoms in cancer patients. The basis of adequate pain control is thorough pain analysis and excellent communication between patient, family and friends, physicians, nurses, and other caregivers. Disease-modifying and symptom-directed therapies are initiated concomitantly and adapted in the course of treatment and disease. Adherence to the WHO guidelines for cancer pain treatment will control pain in the majority of patients. Complicated pain syndromes require a more sophisticated approach, including psychosocial interventions, anesthetic techniques and the entire spectrum of physical methods. Regardless of the existence of validated guidelines, pain therapy requires a highly individualized approach driven by care for the patient.

Nevertheless, complete analgesia might not be the main goal of cancer pain therapy. Within the context of palliative medicine, cancer pain therapy is dedicated to patient rehabilitation, and this means bringing the patient back to the life they desire.

Further reading

Bruera E, Schoeller T, Wenk R et al: A prospective multicenter assessment of the Edmonton staging system for cancer pain. J Pain Symptom Manage 1995; 10: 348–55.

Daut RL, Cleeland CS: The prevalence and severity of pain in cancer. Cancer 1982; 50: 1913–18.

De Stoutz ND, Bruera E, Suarez-Almazor M: Opioid rotation for toxicity reduction in terminal cancer patients. J Pain Symptom Manage 1995; 10: 378–83.

Expert Working Group of the EAPC: Morphine in cancer pain: modes of application. BMJ 1996; 312: 823–6.

Jadad AR: The WHO analgesic ladder for cancer pain management. JAMA 1995; 274: 1870–3.

Ripamonti C, Zecca E, Bruera E: An update on the clinical use of methadone for cancer pain. Pain 1997; 70: 109–15.

Schug SA, Zech D, Dörr U: Cancer pain management according to WHO guidelines. J Pain Symptom Manage 1990; 5: 27–32.

Vainio A, Auvinen A: Prevalence of symptoms among patients with advanced cancer: an international collaborative study. J Pain Symptom Manage 1996; 12: 3–10

Walker VA, Hoskin PJ, Hanks GW, White ID: Evaluation of WHO analgesic guidelines for cancer pain in a hospital-based palliative care unit. J Pain Symptom Manage 1988; 3: 145–9.

World Health Organization: Cancer Pain Relief, 2nd edn. Geneva: WHO, 1997.

Skin problems in advanced cancer

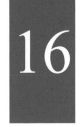

J Lambert, S Rombouts
University Hospital Antwerp, Belgium

Introduction

Dermatological problems occur regularly in advanced cancer care. Pruritus, pressure sores, lymphedema, skin metastasis and fungating wounds are discussed in this chapter.

Pruritus

Types of pruritus

Pruritus or itching can have a peripheral (dermal or neuropathic) or central (neuropathic, neurogenic or psychogenic) origin.

- Itching originating in the skin from inflammation, dryness or other skin damage is termed 'pruritoceptive'.
- If itching arises due to disease at any point along the afferent pathway, it is called neuropathic itching.
- Neurogenic itching originates centrally without evidence of neural disorder. It is often associated with increased opioidergic tone caused by an accumulation of endogenous opioids. Increased serotoninergic tone may also be involved.
- The fourth type of itching is psychogenic.

Causes

Pruritus in patients with advanced cancer may have the following causes:

- dry skin
- malignancies
- drug eruptions
- secondary metabolic effects, such as uremia, cholestasis and paraneoplastic syndromes
- iron deficiency anemia
- acquired ichthyosis.

Hematological disorders

Blood disorders may frequently cause generalized pruritus. In particular, in patients with Hodgkin's disease, polycythemia vera and Sézary's syndrome, itching may be severe. Patients with Waldenström's macroglobinemia, mycosis fungoides, multiple myeloma and leukemia may also have generalized pruritus. The mechanisms in these conditions are poorly understood. Patients with polycythemia vera typically have itching after bathing. The initiating factor seems to be rapid cooling of the skin due to release of pruritogens by granulated mast cells.

Solid tumors

Besides effects such as uremia or cholestasis, almost all of the visceral carcinomas can cause pruritus. The pathogenesis is usually poorly understood. Specific tumors are sometimes associated with localized itch:

- A tumor invading the floor of the fourth ventricle may cause itching or paresthesia localized at the nostrils.
- Scrotal itching may be associated with prostate cancer.
- Perianal itching may be associated with cancers of the sigmoid colon and rectum.
- Vulval itching can be caused by cervical cancer.

Cholestasis

Severe pruritus is a frequent complication of cholestasis. However, not all patients with cholestasis develop pruritus. The reason for this is unknown. Typically, itching starts at the soles of the feet and the palms of the hands, and subsequently becomes more generalized. The pathogenesis of the pruritus may be related to increased opioidergic tone, but the serotoninergic system may also be involved, and itching may be caused by an accumulation of bile salts interacting with nerve endings in the skin.

Uremia

Uremic pruritus is generally classified as mixed, as its complex physiology is unclear because little is known about most of the underlying mechanisms. Many factors appear to be involved. The skin becomes atrophic and dry. Pruritogenic cytokines may be produced in the dermis by various activated cells close to itching receptors. Mast cells are enhanced, possibly in relation to the raised parathyroid hormone plasma concentration that occurs in uremic patients with secondary hyperparathyroidism. There are changes in the relative expression of μ, and κ opioid receptors on lymphocytes. The imbalance in the expression of the opioid receptor subtypes may contribute to the pathogenesis of uremic itching.

Drugs

Many drugs can cause pruritus and drug eruptions, which are in most cases pruritic. Generalized itching occurs in about 1% of patients who are treated with oral, subcutaneous or intravenous opioids and in 10–90% who receive spinal opioids perioperatively. The incidence depends on the type of opioid and whether the patient is opioid-naive.

When injected intradermally, some opioids (morphine and methadone) can cause local itching and a typical histamine weal-and-flare response. Intradermal fentanyl and oxymorphone do not cause this phenomenon.

Histamine release from dermal mast cells is not responsible for itching induced by clinical doses of opioids administered spinally or systematically. In these circumstances, itching may be relieved by naloxone, but not by H_1-antihistamines. Other neurotransmitter systems interact with the opioid system in relation to the mediation of itching, notably the serotonin system. It has recently been suggested that the μ opioid receptors mediate itching, whereas the κ opioid receptors may suppress it.

Treatment

Skin care

Skin care is an essential part of treatment, but is often neglected. Many patients do not require drug treatment if appropriate skin care is given.

■ Adequate nutrition is essential to maintain a healthy skin. The diet should include proteins, carbohydrates, fats, vitamins, minerals and at least 2 liters of fluid a day.

■ The most important aspect is ensuring that the skin does not become dry. Soap must be avoided and replaced by bath or shower oils or fatty soaps. Regular use of emollients is strongly indicated. Emollients soothe, smooth and hydrate the skin. When the skin becomes dry, the balance of skin lipids is reduced, leading to further fluid loss from the skin surface and the increased penetration of skin irritants and allergens. The use of an emollient is essential to restore normal skin balance. Any lotion or cream applied to the skin should be stored in a refrigerator, as this enhances the cooling effect on application.

- Heat should be avoided, as it increases cutaneous blood flow and may enhance itching. Cool temperature lowers the itching threshold. Patients are advised to wear light, cool clothes, to maintain a cool ambient environment that is not too dry, and to avoid alcohol and hot or spicy foods and drinks. Patients are advised to have short, tepid showers or baths, and to dry skin gently by patting with a soft towel. Talcum powder and perfumed deodorants should be avoided, as they contain ingredients that can exacerbate itching. Patients must try not to scratch but to rub gently or apply pressure on the itching part. Applying a cold cloth or ice can help break the itch–scratch–itch cycle.
- Patients must keep fingers nails short and clean, to cause as little damage as possible to the skin.

Drug treatment

Cholestasis

The treatment ladder for itching due to cholestasis is as follows:

- *Step 1:* stenting of common bile duct.
- *Step 2:* naltrexone 12.5–250 mg, once daily (this is contraindicated in patients needing opioids for pain relief) or α-17-alkylandrogen, (e.g. methyltestosterone 25 mg sublingually once daily or danazole 200 mg thrice daily).
- *Step 3:* rifampicin 75 mg once daily to 150 mg twice daily. Rifampicin is not only a hepatic enzyme inducer, but also inhibits bile acid reuptake by hepatocytes and thereby increases plasma bile acid concentrations. However, by interrupting the enteropathic circulation of bile acids, rifampicin may reduce the impact of increased bile acids on the metabolic processes of the liver. To reduce the risk of hepatic dysfunction, it is advisable to start with a low dose. If this is not effective after a week, the dose should be increased to 150 mg once daily and then to 150 mg twice daily.
- *Step 4:* replace with or add colestyramine 4 g × 2 once or twice daily. Colestyramine interrupts the enteral hepatic circulation of bile acids by chelating them in the intestines. It is not effective in itching associated with complete large-duct biliary obstruction. The 4 g sachet is given before and after breakfast, so that the arrival of the resin in the duodenum coincides with gall-bladder contraction. If necessary, a further dose can be taken before the midday and evening meals. The maintenance dose is generally 12 g per day. If used long term, it can cause malabsorption of fat-soluble vitamins.

Ondansetron, a serotonin type 3 receptor (5-HT_3) antagonist, is rather controversial for treatment of pruritus in cholestasis. Excellent results have been reported in case reports and from open-label studies of either single or multiple doses of intravenous and/or oral treatment in chronic cholestasis. However, in randomized controlled trials, there was either no or minimal benefit.

Uremia

The treatment ladder for itching due to uremia is as follows:

- *Step 1:* UVB phototherapy, particularly narrow-band UVB.
- *Step 2:* naltrexone 50–100 mg once nightly. The conflicting trial results are confusing. It is contraindicated in patients needing opioids for pain relief.
- *Step 3:* thalidomide 100 mg once nightly. It is effective in more than 50% of patients.
- *Step 4:* mirtazapine 7.5–15 mg once daily. It is a norepinephrine and serotonin reuptake inhibitor with H_1 antihistamine properties.

Solid tumors

Paraneoplastic itching associated with solid tumors is not eased by corticosteroids or cimetidine. Paroxetine is almost always beneficial, often within 24 hours.

The treatment ladder for itching due to solid tumors is as follows:

- *Step 1:* paroxetine 5–20 mg once daily.
- *Step 2:* mirtazapine 7.5–15 mg once nightly.
- *Step 3:* combination of paroxetine and mirtazapine.
- *Step 4:* Thalidomide 100 mg once nightly.

Paroxetine is a selective serotonin reuptake inhibitor (SSRI). Two hypotheses are considered to explain paroxetine's antipruritic activity:

- Chronic paroxetine therapy may modify central opioid receptors. Acute effects may be related to an increase of serotonin concentration, acting upon the postsynaptic receptors. Stimulation of 5-HT_2 and 5-HT_3 receptors might be responsible for the nausea and vomiting observed in the paroxetine responders during the first days of therapy. The effect is short-lasting, and ondansetron, a 5-HT_3 receptor antagonist, is used to control the nausea.
- Paroxetine strongly inhibits the CYP2D6 hepatic isoenzyme, which is involved in the metabolism of codeine to morphine. It is possible that this enzyme is involved in the activation of other (opioid) pruritogens.

Hematological diseases

■ Polycythemia vera: the drug of choice for itching is low-dose aspirin: 300 mg is generally effective within 30 minutes for 12–24 hours. Because platelet degranulation is increased in polycythemia and is known to be decreased by aspirin, the antipruritic effect of aspirin could be related to its impact on platelet dynamics.

■ Hodgkin's lymphoma: curative radiotherapy and/or chemotherapy is the best approach in Hodgkin's lymphoma. Corticosteroids often relieve itching in late-stage disease. The mechanism of its effect is unknown. In the case of no effect, cimetidine 800 mg/24 hours or mirtazapine 7.5–15 mg once nightly may be considered.

Opioid-induced itching

Opioid-induced itching is rare in palliative care. Few patients receive spinal opioids, and those who do are not opioid-naive. When itching is induced by a systemic opioid, opiod switching may be helpful (e.g. from morphine to hydromorphone).

Cutaneous tumor involvement
Prevalence

Cutaneous tumor involvement is a result of direct tumor extension by an underlying tumor or by hematogenous or lymphatic dissemination of neoplastic cells. The exact incidence of cutaneous metastasis is unknown, but the skin is an uncommon site of metastatic disease. Large studies suggest an incidence of 5–9%.

In men, primary cancers of the lung and colon are most often seen, whereas in women, breast and colon cancer are more frequent. Carcinomas of the ovary, stomach and kidney are also frequent causes of skin metastasis.

Clinical presentation
Aspect

Most cutaneous metastases present as nonspecific painless dermal or subcutaneous nodules, with an intact overlying epidermis. The most common clinical findings are clusters of discrete, firm, painless nodules emerging rapidly on a given anatomical site, proliferating swiftly and then remaining stationary. Occasionally, cutaneous metastases are as large as a nodule of several centimeters or have a miliary aspect and may even be hardly visible. They may be flesh-colored, pink, violet or brown–black, and are often stony hard. They may appear as multiple small papules, sometimes numbering in the hundreds, as large tumors, as sclerotic plaques or as hemangioma-like nodules. At times, scalp alopecia may be produced (usually from breast cancer). They can also become necrotic and ulcerated. They may resemble cilindromas or pilar cysts (usually in the case of prostate, breast or colon cancer). Metastases may be hyperkeratotic, suggesting a cutaneous horn or a keratoacanthoma. Rarely, metastases may be unilateral (zosteriform) or grow like a cluster of grapes (botryoid).

Several primary cutaneous disorders may be mimicked by cutaneous metastases. Renal cell carcinoma metastases may resemble Kaposi's sarcoma or pyogenic granuloma; lymphoma cutis or a transitional cell carcinoma may resemble a penile chancre.

The growth pattern of skin metastases is unpredictable and may not reflect that of the primary tumor. They may grow rapidly, or they may be slow-growing and solitary.

Metastases may sometimes occur within other cutaneous eruptions or at radiation or surgical sites. Radiation scars may be infiltrated by an underlying radiation-induced malignancy. Skin metastases may result from implantation after a surgical procedure such as a needle biopsy.

Location

The localization of metastatic skin disease does not occur in a completely random fashion.

In 75% of men, localization of secondary tumors is on the skin of the head, neck, anterior chest and abdomen, together accounting for only about 25% of the body surface. In women, approximately 75% are on the cutaneous surface of the anterior chest and abdomen, comprising less than 20% of the skin surface. Metastases of colorectal carcinoma are most often located in abdominal or perineal areas, and tend to appear after the primary cancer has been identified. The abdominal wall is the most common site for tumors presenting as metastatic disease, with lung cancer most frequently seen. About 10% of the metastatic tumors in the abdominal wall affect the umbilicus.

A wide variety of cutaneous metastases occur on the scalp. The primary cancer in men is often in the lung or kidney, and it is frequently an early finding. In women, breast cancer is the most frequent tumor, usually as a late event.

Facial metastases more often are from oral cavity squamous cell carcinomas, hypernephromas, lung cancer and breast cancer.

Eyelid metastases are most often from breast cancer or melanoma. Dissemination through the valveless vertebral venous system, which bypasses the lungs, may account for seemingly unexpected patterns of metastatic spread, such as prostate and breast cancer to the scalp or face.

Cancers may also invade the overlying skin by direct extension. Most neck cutaneous metastases are deep nodules from extension from cervical lymph nodes, with primary tumors most likely in the oral cavity, lung or breast. Metastases to the upper extremities are uncommon, usually late, findings, and they are even less common in the lower extremities. Sometimes, cutaneous metastases may be scattered in various anatomical sites, either early while an underlying tumor is unsuspected or as a late distant metastasis. Skin metastases are relatively often identified before a primary tumor in the lung or kidney, because early venous invasion through channels including the vertebral venous system may take the metastasis to a distant site. The cutaneous metastasis may provide an opportunity for an early diagnosis. Nevertheless, skin metastases still have a poor prognosis, especially in patients with cancer of the lung, ovary, upper respiratory tract or upper digestive tract. Most patients with umbilical metastasis die within months of detection.

Because carcinoma of the breast is both a common cancer in women and one often involving the skin, and patients with hematological malignancies are especially predisposed to the development of skin lesions associated with their disease, these two disorders are discussed in detail.

Breast carcinoma

Breast carcinoma has eight distinct clinicopathological types of cutaneous involvement. These patterns are not restricted to breast cancer, but rather are probably most evident because of the commonness of breast cancer itself and because of its cutaneous infiltrations.

1. Inflammatory metastatic carcinoma or carcinoma erysipelatoides is characterized by an erythematous patch or plaque with an active spreading border resembling erysipelas, usually affecting the breast and nearby skin. However, other sites can be involved solely, such as the forearm. Rarely, metastases from other carcinomas may produce this clinical pattern. The clinical appearance of inflammation is caused by capillary congestion. There are tumor cells within dilated lymphatics and no acute inflammatory infiltrate.
2. En cuirasse metastatic carcinoma is characterized by a diffuse, morphea-like induration of the skin. It is rare, but is also seen in patients

with lung, gastrointestinal tract, kidney and other metastasizing malignancies. It usually begins as scattered, firm, lenticular papulonodules overlying an erythematous or red–blue, smooth, cutaneous surface. These papulonodules coalesce into a sclerodermoid plaque with no associated inflammatory changes.

3. Teleangiectactic metastatic carcinoma is characterized by violaceous papulovesicles, resembling lymphangioma circumscriptum.

4. The nodular form of metastatic carcinoma usually appears as multiple firm papulonodules or nodules. Occasionally, it may be solitary; a few may be ulcerated or rarely bullous.

5. Alopecia neoplastica, unlike the previous four types, is probably caused by hematogenous rather than lymphatic spread. It appears as painless, nonpruritic, well-demarcated, oval plaques, often displaying a red–pink tone and a smooth surface, resembling alopecia areata.

6. Paget's disease of the breast represents a distinct pattern of cutaneous infiltration from breast cancer and displays a specific histological pattern. It is a sharply demarcated plaque or patch of erythema and scaling, occurring on the nipple or areola, associated with an underlying breast cancer.

7. Breast cancer of the inframammary crease appears as a cutaneous exophytic nodule, clinically suggestive of a primary cutaneous squamous or basal cell carcinoma. It often occurs in women with pendulous breasts and resembles an intertriginous dermatitis or a callus. It may be overlooked.

8. Metastatic mammary carcinoma of the eyelid with hystiocytoid histology is rare and presents as painless eyelid swelling with induration or nodularity, or occasionally as a discrete nodule.

Hematological disorders

Skin lesions that accompany systemic leukemia or lymphoma may contain malignant cells (specific lesions), or they may represent a benign dermatosis that results from either systemic effects of the disease or paraneoplastic phenomena (nonspecific lesions). It is estimated that 25–40% of patients exhibit cutaneous manifestations during the course of their disease. Most often, these are nonspecific lesions, such as Sweet's syndrome, leukocytoclastic vasculitis or ichthyosis.

Some of these signs and symptoms suggest a particular underlying disorder: pruritus, ichthyosis and pigmentary changes frequently occur in Hodgkin's lymphoma, and pallor and ecchymoses are common in acute leukemia.

Specific lesions, termed 'leukemia cutis' or 'lymphoma cutis', may have a variety of appearances, but they often resemble carcinomatous cutaneous metastases and appear as firm papules, nodules or plaques. Individual lesions are more likely to be hemorrhagic or plum-colored, and they may be confused with sarcoidosis, benign lymphocytic infiltration, insect bite reaction or secondary syphilis.

The distribution of lesions sometimes provides a clue to the type of associated malignancy, because lesions on the extremities and face tend to be seen with acute leukemia and chronic lymphocytic leukemia, whereas truncal lesions suggest chronic myeloid leukemia.

Oral lesions, especially hypertrophy and bleeding of the gingivae, are particularly common in monocytic leukemia.

Extramedullarly collections of malignant plasma cells occur in up to 70% of patients with multiple myeloma, but cutaneous plasmacytomas are uncommon.

Lymphedema

Lymphedema is a chronic condition, caused by the abnormal accumulation of a protein-rich fluid in the interstitial space, due to inadequate lymphatic drainage.

Clinical manifestations include swelling, fibrosis and hardening of affected tissues, leading to decreased joint mobility, pain and discomfort. The static, protein-rich environment promotes bacteria, increasing the risk of infection.

Estimates of the incidence of breast-cancer-related lymphedema range from 6% to 83%. Edema may arise immediately or many years after treatment. A wide variety of risk factors have been described: trauma to the lymphatic system, soft-tissue infection, weight gain after treatment, vein puncture in the ipsilateral arm, axillary node status, number of axillary nodes removed, surgical procedure and age. In one prospective study, skin puncture during hospitalization, mastectomy and body mass index (BMI) over 26 were the only significant risk factors.

Multilayered compression bandaging is a primary treatment option in reducing arm lymphedema volume. Further studies are needed to evaluate the additional benefit of manual lymph drainage and hyperbaric oxygen therapy.

Pressure sores

Many patients with advanced cancer are at high risk of developing pressure sores. Prolonged immobilization, circulatory disturbances and poor nutrition are important risk factors.

Etiology

Pressure is the most important etiological factor in ulcer formation. External pressure is generally concentrated over bony prominences. High pressure raises interstitial pressure, compromising oxygenation and microcirculation. There is an inverse time/pressure curve, with slow ulcer formation at low occlusive pressure and rapid ulcer formation at high pressure. When a patient lies on a hospital mattress, pressures of 150 mmHg can be generated. A constant pressure of 70 mmHg for 2 hours leads to tissue death. If, however, pressure is intermittently relieved, minimal changes occur. The duration as well as degree of pressure is important. The highest interstitial pressures occur at the bone/muscle interface, with less damage at the dermoepidermal level. Deep tissue trauma can occur with relatively little superficial damage.

Externally applied pressure alone is more effective than shear in reducing skin arteriolar blood flow, but vascular occlusion is particularly enhanced if both factors are combined.

Shearing forces are major contributors to the size and grade of pressure ulcers. They result from the sliding and relative displacement of two apposing surfaces. When the head of a patient is raised more than 30%, shearing forces occur in the sacral and coccygeal areas.

Sliding of the torso transmits pressure to the sacrum and deep fascia, although the outer sacral skin is fixed because of friction with the bed.

Friction also reduces the amount of pressure needed to produce ulcers. Friction is the force that resists relative motion between two contact surfaces. It results when a bedridden patient is dragged across the bed sheets. The protective stratum corneum is damaged, the skin barrier is compromised and skin ulceration is enhanced.

A long-term moist environment resulting from perspiration or fecal or urinary incontinence can increase the risk of pressure ulcer formation by fivefold.

Risk factors

Besides etiological factors, several risk factors may further predispose to the development of pressure ulcers, namely, prolonged immobilization and sensory deficit that impedes the ability to perceive pain resulting from prolonged pressure. Circulatory disturbances causing poor oxygen perfusion, such as anemia, blood dyscrasia or interstitial edema, may also enhance skin ulceration, as well as delay healing.

Pressure ulcers developed in 75% of patients with low serum albumin levels (<3.5 g/dl) versus 16.6% of patients with normal levels. Malnutrition leads to reduction in subcutaneous fat and delay in wound healing. The development and severity of pressure ulcers seem to correlate with the extent of malnutrition. Dry skin, smoking, sedatives and analgesics, which reduce pain sensation and mobility, are additional risk factors.

To identify persons at risk so that preventive measures can be implemented, several risk assessment tools have been proposed, such as the Braden Scale and the Norton Scale.

Complications

Infection can complicate pressure ulcers. It is important to make a distinction between bacterial colonization and bacterial infection.

Colonization refers to the harmless presence of microorganisms. Most wounds are colonized. Even when they are heavily colonized, healing occurs in the majority of these wounds. Clinically, there are no signs of infection.

Infection is easily recognized by the presence of surrounding redness, heat and pain. Purulent discharge, foul odor and systemic signs may also be present. In some patients, infection can be unapparent. Patients frequently have other medical problems such as decreased sensation, disturbed immunological response or abnormal neurological function. Pain, fever and leukocytosis may not be prominent. Pressure ulcers can cause bacteremia. The prognosis is poor, and the course may be complicated by sepsis, endocarditis and death.

Most pressure ulcers are not associated with osteomyelitis. In nonhealing pressure ulcers, however, an underlying bone infection occurs in approximately one-third of cases. Osteomyelitis can occur through direct extension or through blood dissemination. In long-lasting pressure ulcers, well-differentiated squamous cell carcinoma can occur. It usually behaves aggressively, with a metastatis rate of approximately 61%.

Sinus tracts frequently occur even in pressure ulcers that seem to be superficial. These may extend deep enough to reach the joint space and cause osteomyelitis. A sinogram is useful in determining the extent of surgical debridement. Pressure sores may communicate with deep viscera, such as the bowel and bladder.

Prevention

- Prevention can reduce the incidence of pressure ulcers by at least 50%. Preventive measures must be focused on patients at risk. For those patients, a skin inspection should be performed at least once daily, with particular attention to bony prominences. The skin must be kept clean, well hydrated and free of excess moisture.
- Massaging bony prominences has no proven benefit and indeed may lead to deep tissue damage.
- Friction and shear can be minimized by lifting rather than dragging the patient off a bed or wheelchair; and by keeping the bed free of particulate matter, such as food crumbs, and loose sheets that limit restriction of movement. Elevating the head of the bed more than 30° should be avoided to limit undue pressure on the ischial tuberosity and calcaneus.
- Pressure relief is probably the most important factor in preventing pressure ulcers. All bedridden patients should have a pressure-relieving mattress in addition to frequent repositioning. A patient should be turned at least every 2 hours. Soft pillows or foam wedges can be used for support and to prevent bony prominences, such as ankles or knees, from direct contact with one another.
- The general medical condition of the patient should be monitored, and particular attention should be paid to nutrition.

Wound management

- (Surgical) removal of necrotic debris from the wound surface is needed to allow granulation tissue formation and re-epithelialization. Depending on the ulceration, surgical debridement, moist dressings 2–3 times a day, occlusive dressings or enzymatic debridement will be preferred.
- It is important to keep the wound clean and free of infection.
- For adequate follow-up and management, the ulcer should be assessed at least once a week and the presence of sinus tracts, undermining, tunneling, necrotic tissue, exudate, granulation tissue and epithelialization documented.
- Wound occlusion promotes re-epithelialization, reduces associated pain, enhances autolytic debridement and provides a barrier to bacteria. In most patients, a dressing that provides moist wound healing is used. A variety of dressings, each with its own indication, are on the market.
- In some patients, surgical reconstruction will be needed.
- Other treatment options are growth factors and cultured keratinocyte grafts and skin substitutes.

Fungating wounds

The term 'fungating wound' is often used interchangeably with the term 'malignant lesions'. Both terms refer to the infiltration and proliferation of malignant cells through the epidermis of the skin. The tumors may be locally advanced, metastatic or recurrent. Any tumor can result in a fungating wound, and tumor progression through the skin follows diverse patterns. Fungating breast cancer presents in a number of ways, such as deep necrotic ulceration with proliferative growth of the ulcer margins or extensive cutaneous infiltration of the chest wall. Carcinomas of the rectum and genitourinary tract can cause protruding perineal growth, gross deformity and loss of normal function, which may include fistulae involving the bladder, vagina and bowel. Carcinomas of the ovary, cecum and rectum, which infiltrate the anterior wall of the abdomen, may present initially as small raised nodules that develop into necrotic, cauliflower-like structures. Head and neck tumors may communicate with the buccal cavity.

Tissue hypoxia can present a significant problem, as anaerobic organisms flourish in accessible necrotic tissue, which is a characteristic of most fungating tumors. The malodorous volatile fatty acids, a metabolic end product, are responsible for the characteristic smell and profuse exudate that is often associated with fungating wounds.

The major problems include pain, soreness and irritation of excoriated skin conditions, pruritus, odor, spontaneous bleeding, and hemorrhage.

The pruritus is a creeping, intense itching sensation attributed to the activity of the tumor. It is generally not responsive to antihistamines. Hormone therapy or palliative chemotherapy can help.

Three main approaches are possible for the management of odor:

- Systemic antibiotics are used to reduce bacterial colonization and control the offensive odor from volatile metabolic end products.
- Topical metronidazole is an alternative if systemic therapy is not recommended.
- Activated charcoal dressings act as filters to absorb the volatile malodorous chemicals from the wound before they pass into the air. They are useless, however, when they cannot be fitted as a sealed unit.

Oral antifibrinolytics, radiotherapy and embolization are used to control spontaneous bleeding from eroding blood vessels.

Besides these special problems, the principles of wound healing must be followed.

Further reading

Bosonnet L: Pruritis: scratching the surface. Eur J Cancer Care 2003; 12: 162–5.

Clark B, Sitzia J, Harlow W: Incidence and risk of arm oedema following treatment for breast cancer: a three-year follow-up study. Q J Med 2005; 98: 343–8.

Grocott P, Cowley S: The palliative management of fungating malignant wounds – generalising from multiple-case study data using a system of reasoning. Int J Nurs Stud 2001; 38: 533–46.

Kanj LF, Wilking SVB, Phillips T: Pressure ulcers. J Am Acad Dermatol 1998; 38: 517–36.

Schwartz RA: Cutaneous metastatic disease. J Am Acad Dermatol 1995; 33: 161–82.

Twycross R, Greaves MW, Handwerker H et al: Itch: scratching more than the surface. Q J Med 2003; 96: 7–26.

17 Other problems

Y Yildirim, O Ozyilkan
Baskent University, Turkey

Hiccup

Prevalence

The incidence of hiccup in patients with cancer has not been studied, but is estimated to be 1–9%. Hiccup is more frequent among male patients.

Hiccup is usually short-lived and uncomplicated. It can occur anywhere between 2 and 60 times a minute. Common causes of hiccup are presented in Table 17.1. Chronic hiccup is defined as attacks that are recurrent and persist longer than 48 hours. Intractable hiccup is rarely seen in patients with cancer; about 100 cases have been presented in the literature. It is a distressing symptom that may be associated with insomnia, depression, weakness and weight loss.

Pathophysiology

Hiccup is a complex pathological reflex that consists of involuntary, spasmodic and short-lasting contractions of the diaphragm associated with

Table 17.1 Common causes of hiccup

Central nervous system disorders: closed head trauma, skull fractures, meningitis, encephalitis, tumors
Mass lesions: goiters, aneurysm, diverticula, mediastinal tumors, lung, gastric or esophageal cancer
Gastric distention: hepatomegaly
Diaphragmatic irritation: abscess, cholecystitis, pleurisy
Irritative stimuli: gastroesophageal reflux, spicy food, gastritis, peptic ulcer
Metabolic disorders: hyponatremia, hypocalcemia, hypocapnia, hyperuremia
Drugs: dexamethasone, methylprednisolone, diazepam, midazolam, barbiturates, etoposide

sudden closure of the glottis after the beginning of inspiratory flow. The pathway of the hiccup reflex arc is composed of afferent fibers, a central part and efferent branches. The afferent pathway contains the vagal, phrenic and sympathetic nerve branches at T6–T12. The central part originates between the C3 and C5 cervical segments of the spinal cord, and is probably linked to the supratentorial area and hypothalamus. The efferent limb consists of the phrenic nerve to the diaphragm and nerves to the glottis and intercostal muscles.

Treatment

Initial management of hiccup includes evaluation of possible causes. Particular attention should be given to any medication (dexamethasone, barbiturates, diazepam or others) that causes hiccup. Cessation of these treatments should be considered whenever possible. Hiccup induced by a stomach compressed due to hepatomegaly may be controlled by metoclopramide (10 mg/day).

Other symptomatic treatments are:

- Chlorpromazine (10–25 mg/day) however, physicians should be aware of the increased incidence of adverse effects of chlorpromazine, such as sedation, postural hypotension and xerostomia (in older patients).
- Baclofen, a γ-aminobutyric acid (GABA) derivative with presynaptic motor neuron inhibitor properties at the spinal level and postsynaptic inhibitory properties, has been found to be effective in intractable hiccup. Baclofen (5–10 mg twice or thrice daily up to 20 mg/day) can suppress hiccup when other agents have failed. However, adverse effects of baclofen may be observed at dosages of 80 mg or more. Treatment should be discontinued slowly to avoid withdrawal symptoms (tachycardia, hallucinations and convulsions).
- Other drugs include haloperidol (1.5–3 mg intramuscularly), valproic acid (up to 15 mg/day in divided doses) and nefopam (10 mg intravenously). Midazolam, nifedipine, carbamazepine, diphenylhydantoin, gabapentin and methylphenidate have also been tried in the management of intractable hiccup.
- Cervical nerve blockage is the final resort in patients with hiccup resistant to all other medical therapies.

Bleeding

Hemorrhagic problems associated with malignancy are common in oncology practice. Awareness and preventive measures have markedly decreased the incidence of death from hemorrhage in patients with cancer in recent years.

Thrombocytopenia

Thrombocytopenia is one of the most common causes of bleeding in this population. Various pathophysiological events, including bone-marrow infiltration, infections and cancer therapy, may cause thrombocytopenia.

Petechiae are characteristic of severe thrombocytopenia. Ecchymoses and subcutaneous collection of blood are the typical physical findings. The most common sites of bleeding are the skin and mucous membranes.

Recently, clinical guidelines have been determined for platelet transfusion in patients with cancer. Platelet counts of $10\,000/\mu l$ or lower may be associated with severe bleeding. Prophylactic platelet transfusion for patients at this threshold is recommended. However, a threshold platelet count of $20\,000/\mu l$ may be considered for patients receiving aggressive treatment for bladder cancer as well as those with demonstrated necrotic tumors, or for patients with acute leukemia and accompanying signs of hemorrhage, high fever, hyperleukocytosis, rapid fall of platelet count or coagulation problems. Recombinant interleukin-11 (IL-11) appears to shorten the duration of thrombocytopenia and may result in a decrease in bleeding only in patients with chemotherapy-induced thrombocytopenia. The platelet count should be maintained above $40\,000$–$50\,000/\mu l$ if there is a possibility of a surgical or invasive procedure.

Immune thrombocytopenia

Immune thombocytopenia may occur in lymphoproliferative disorders. Treatment with intravenous immune globulin at a dosage of 1 g/kg/day for 2 days or prednisone (1 mg/kg/day for 2 weeks followed by a gradual decrease) can be effective.

Vitamin K deficiency

Vitamin K deficiency is another common cause of bleeding. Cancer-induced anorexia and malnutrition or concomitant use of antibiotics results in vitamin K deficiency. Prothrombin time is prolonged. Administration of vitamin K at a dosage of 10 mg/day (orally, subcutaneously or intravenously for 3–5 days) is recommended.

Diffuse intravascular coagulation (DIC)

Life-threatening bleeding can be a clinical presentation of disseminated intravascular coagulation (DIC), observed frequently in malignancies and major infections.

In most cases (other than severe mucousal hemorrhage), bleeding from surgical incisions, venipuncture or catheter sites may be observed. In patients with cancer, chronic DIC may present as abnormalities in laboratory analyses, with no clinical signs. Occasionally, DIC may present as thrombosis.

The diagnosis of DIC is suspected in patients with thrombocytopenia, microangiopathic hemolytic anemia, prolonged prothrombin time (PT), partial thromboplastin time (PTT) and thrombin time, and elevated fibrin degradation products. However, the most comprehensive diagnostic test for DIC is the D-dimer immunoassay that measures fibrin derivatives. Fibrinogen levels decrease in DIC, and low levels are associated with severe bleeding.

Treatment depends on the underlying causes, and reversible factors should be corrected immediately. Platelet transfusion and fresh frozen plasma replacement can be performed in patients with bleeding. The addition of heparin is not indicated and should be reserved for patients with thrombosis. ε-Aminocaproic acid or tranexamic acid can be considered in severe bleeding.

Sweating
Prevalence

Sweating is a distressing symptom that may result in deterioration of a patient's quality of life or a decrease in social interaction or daily activities. It can be generalized, involving the whole body, or focal, involving a limited area of the body (most commonly, armpits, hands, feet, hands or face). Generalized sweating can be part of underlying disease (e.g. myeloproliferative disorders, Hodgkin's lymphoma), or endocrine disorders (hyperthyroidism, hyperpituitarism, diabetes mellitus, pheochromocytoma or carcinoid syndrome), infections, cardiovascular shock, drugs (antiestrogens, antiandrogens, opioids, tricyclic antidepressants and corticosteroids), and menopause (natural or surgically, or chemotherapy- or radiotherapy-induced). Paraneoplastic tumor-induced fever can be another cause of sweating in cancer patients.

The actual incidence of sweating in patients with cancer is not known. It differs with tumor type and stage of the disease. In patients with advanced cancer, the prevalence of sweating is 14–28% and it occurs mostly at night.

Sweating, sometimes together with hot flushes, is a troublesome symptom in survivors of breast cancer. Approximately 12–14% of patients with breast cancer treated with antiestrogens experience sweating as an adverse effect. More than half of patients with prostate cancer may have similar symptoms due to androgen-depleting therapy.

Treatment

Treatment of sweating consists of management of the underlying causes and palliation of the symptom. Attention should be paid to drugs used in cancer therapy or palliation, as many of these may have sweating as an adverse effect.

■ Opioid-induced sweating usually does not respond to opioid switch. It can be controlled by nonsteroidal anti-inflammatory drugs (NSAIDs). Antimuscarinic drugs may be effective. Low-dose thioridazine has been found to be effective in this indication. Olanzapine, a new antipsychotic agent, can control opioid-induced sweating.

■ Sweating due to tumor-induced fever can be controlled by NSAIDs. Some reports indicate that thalidomide is effective in controlling sweats caused by tumor-induced fever.

■ Somatostatin analogs are effective for controlling symptoms of neuroendocrine tumors and may be useful in nonspecific management of sweating.

■ In patients with breast or prostate cancer, sweating and hot flushes can be treated with low-dose megestrol acetate and selective serotonin reuptake inhibitors (SSRIs). Megesterol acetate at a dosage of 20 mg orally twice daily has been found to decrease symptoms within 3 weeks. Venlafaxine is another drug used to manage sweating. Compared with megestrol acetate, its effect is observed rapidly, usually within days. To avoid adverse effects, venlafaxine should be started at a dose of 37.5 mg/day and increased to the optimal dosage, namely 75 mg/day. Many alternative and complementary interventions have been tried to reduce symptoms.

Prevention and treatment of thromboembolic complications

Prevalence

Cancer is a well-known cause of prothrombosis and is associated with increased venous and arterial thrombosis. Cancer patients constitute 15–20% of all patients with thromboembolic events. Cancer increases the risk of venous thromboembolism (VTE) by 4–6 times. The overall incidence of

Table 17.2 *Intrinsic and extrinsic factors promoting the coagulation system*

Intrinsic factors:
Tissue factor (TF)-like procoagulant: leukemia, lymphoma, adenocarcinomas, osteogenic sarcomas
Cancer procoagulant (CP, a vitamin-K-dependent cysteine protease that directly activates factor X): sarcoma, neuroblastoma, melanoma, lung, breast, colon, kidney and vaginal cancer, hematological malignancies
Other prothrombotic factors: cancer-produced mucin and factor V receptor expression
Cytokines released by tumor or host cells increase platelet aggregation and activation
Increased activity of plasminogen activator inhibitor 1 (PAT-1); decreased plasma levels of antithrombin III and natural anticoagulants
Endothelial cells become procoagulant owing to inflammatory cytokines, particularly tumor necrosis factor (TNF) and interleukin-1 (IL-1)
Extrinsic factors:
Chemotherapy: high-dose chemotherapy in bone-marrow transplantation
l-asparaginase and tamoxifen
Radiotherapy
Surgery
Central venous catheterization
Immobilization

clinically significant thrombosis is 5–60% in different malignancies. The most common malignancies complicated by thrombosis are lung and pancreatic cancers in men, and gynecological, pancreatic and colorectal cancers in women. Multiple intrinsic and extrinsic factors that promote coagulation have been described in different malignancies (Table 17.2).

Diagnosis

Leg swelling, pain and erythema, together with elevated levels of D-dimers, can be a sensitive screen for suspected VTE.

■ Duplex ultrasound with compression is a sensitive and specific diagnostic procedure for lower-extremity VTE.

- Many patients with catheter-related upper extremity thrombosis might be asymptomatic. Symptoms may include swelling and pain in the arm and face, as well as headache.
- Contrast venography is the reference standard for diagnosis of upper-extremity thrombosis.
- Chest pain, hemoptysis, dyspnea and hypoxia are the major signs of pulmonary embolism (PE). Ventilation–perfusion scintigraphy is highly specific in the diagnosis of PE. Although pulmonary contrast angiography is the reference standard, it is of limited use. Computed tomography (CT) angiogram and spiral CT are useful in differential diagnosis.

Treatment

- Initial treatment of acute VTE starts with heparin, either low-molecular weight heparin (LMWH) or unfractionated heparin (UFH), followed by a coumarin derivative (e.g. warfarin).
- LMWH and UFH have similar efficacies, and clinical trials have shown that the use of LMWH without monitoring is as safe as UFH.
- Warfarin is the standard for secondary prophylaxis. However, many drugs and chemotherapeutic agents in gastrointestinal and liver disorders may alter the anticoagulant response to warfarin. Regular evaluation of the International Normalized Ratio (INR) is needed to adjust the anticoagulant response.
- Recently, dalteparin, a LMWH, has been found to be effective and safe as a secondary prophylaxis of VTE.
- Catheter-related thrombosis is treated with fibrinolytic agents (tissue-type plasminogen activator (tPA), streptokinase or urokinase). Pre-existing clotting defects, bleeding source, central nervous system metastasis, recent major surgery, and a history of gastrointestinal bleeding or uncontrolled hypertension are contraindications to thrombolytic treatment.
- In cases of extensive thrombosis or multiple PE, thrombolytic treatments must be followed by heparin and warfarin. Warfarin should be continued for the duration of catheter use and for 3 months after removal of the catheter.

Prevention

Primary prevention is advisable in patients with cancer who undergo surgery. With the use of UFH or LMWH, a 80% reduction in the risk of thromboembolic events has been observed.

Furthermore, LMWH therapy in advanced cancer patients has been found to improve survival. Results are promising for antithrombolytic therapy and its effect on cancer mortality; further studies are highly recommended.

Further reading

Lee AYY: Management of thrombosis in cancer: primary prevention and secondary prophylaxis. Br J Haematol 2004; 128: 291–302.

Ripamonti C, Fusco F: Respiratory problems in advanced cancer. Support Care Cancer 2002; 10: 204–16.

Schiffer CA, Anderson KC, Bennelt CL et al: Platelet transfusion for patients with cancer: clinical practice guidelines of the American Society of Clinical Oncology. J Clin Oncol 2001; 19: 1519–38.

Sutherland DE, Weitz IC, Leibmen HA: Thromboembolic complications of cancer: epidemiology, pathogenesis, diagnosis, and treatment. Am J Hematol 2003; 72: 43–52.

Zhukovsky DS: Fever and sweats in the patients with advanced cancer. Hematol Oncol Clin North Am 2002; 16: 579–88.

18 Geriatric patients with advanced cancer

M Wagnerová
East Slovak Oncology Institute, Slovak Republic

Introduction

Cancer is primarily a disease of the elderly, in whom its incidence and mortality rates are high. The definition of 'elderly' is a highly individualized process. The typical division of populations into older or younger than 65 years is often used in the medical literature. Studies further categorize patients as older than 75 years, and social gerontologists have coined the term 'oldest old' for those 85 years old and older. Geriatricians have introduced the Comprehensive Geriatric Assessment (CGA) for classifying patients by their physiological rather than chronological age. Cancer is a major public health problem that disproportionately affects older persons.

Incidence and mortality

Persons older than 65 years are a growing percentage of the US and European populations currently around 13–18% and expected to increase to almost 20% by 2030. The number of persons older than 65 years was approximately 35 million in 2000, and is likely to double to 70 million by 2050.

Cancer mortality is highest in the elderly, with 70% of all deaths due to malignant disease being in persons aged 65 years or older. The incidence of cancer in elderly men and women is 11 times higher than that in younger persons. Elderly patients account for a large part of the expected increase in the number of persons with cancer: from 1.3 million in 2000 to 2.6 million in 2050. The number of cases in persons aged 75 years and older is expected almost to triple between 2000 and 2050.

The lifetime risk of cancer is higher in men than in women (559.6 per 100 000 vs 420.1 per 100 000). Lung cancer is the most common fatal cancer in both men and women older than 60 years. In the age group 60–79 years, the second and the third ranked fatal malignant diseases in women are breast and colorectal cancer, in men they are colorectal cancer and prostate cancer. Since 1970, the incidence of nonmelanoma skin cancer, non-Hodgkin's lymphoma and malignant brain tumors has dramatically increased in the elderly. The causes of this increase are not clear, and it could be that age-related molecular changes make older persons more susceptible to environmental carcinogenesis.

Evaluation

Older patients have highly variable physiological ages, and their diagnostics and treatment should be individualized for optimal outcomes. Treatment paradigms should also take into account

- the diversity of patient life expectancy
- functional reserve
- social support
- personal preference.

The relatively poor outcomes in older patients may be due in part to undertreatment – whether from lack of treatment or the use of substandard doses and regimens. Undertreatment may result from the persistent belief that elderly patients cannot tolerate the toxicities of standard treatment. Chronological age should not be a barrier to the use of potentially curative therapy or palliative, life-prolonging treatment: studies have shown that, with appropriate supportive care, otherwise healthy older patients can obtain the same benefit from standard treatment as younger patients.

The elderly are highly diverse in terms of comorbidity. One way to account for this diversity was proposed by Hamerman (Table 18.1). This system reflects the life expectancy and the functional reserve of older individuals, and thus may be useful to plan individualized cancer treatment.

Table 18.1 Staging of older people according to the potential for intervention and clinical correlates

Primary group	Complete independence	Coping
Intermediate group	Partial independence	Functional decline Coping with difficulty
Secondary group	Frailty	Disability Failure to cope
Tertiary group	Dependence	Near death

A multidimensional assessment is a key part of the treatment approach for older patients in a geriatric setting. Comorbidity, functional status, depression, cognitive impairment, nutritional status and insufficient social support have all been demonstrated to affect the survival of elderly cancer patients, with a relative risk of death.

In 1996, a CGA scale was developed and validated for the first time in an oncology setting by Monfardini and colleagues. The CGA is routinely employed in geriatric clinics, but is not yet widely used by oncologists.

Geriatric assessment may serve as a predictor of clinical outcome and a research tool through which one may learn more about the biology and treatment of cancer in older people. The CGA scale has not been standardized, and the consensus is that it should include the elements listed in Table 18.2.

Treatment

For optimal treatment choice, the following additional factors need to be considered.

Tumor-related factors
- malignancy type
- estimated survival without treatment
- availability of effective treatments
- morbidity associated with treatment.

Patient-related factors
- age and estimated survival independent of the effect of existing malignancy
- fitness for therapy, as estimated by geriatric assessment
- patient desires
- other social factors, including family desires and travel resources
- economic resources.

Surgery

Surgery is still the most important treatment for solid tumors, irrespective of age. Nevertheless, elderly patients have a higher potential operative risk of morbidity and mortality due to the presence of comorbidity and physiological reduction of functional reserve connected to aging. For example, elderly patients are more sensitive than younger patients to volume depletions that

Table 18.2 Elements of a comprehensive geriatric assessment

Factor	Tools for assessment	Other assessments
Functional status	Activities of Daily Living (ADL); Instrumental Activities of Daily Living (IADL); Performance status	
Comorbidity	Charlson Comorbidity Index; Cumulative Illness Rating Scale–Geriatrics (CIRS-G)	
Socioeconomic issues		Living conditions; caregiver presence and competence; income; access to transportation
Nutritional status	Mini Nutritional Assessment (MNA)	
Polypharmacy		Number of medications; drug–drug interactions
Geriatric syndromes	Geriatric Depression Scale (GDS); Folstein Mini Mental Status	Delirium; falls; osteoporosis; neglect and abuse; failure to thrive

are often associated with wide resections and longer surgical procedures typical of surgical oncology, and less resistant to postoperative infections due to the progressive impairment of the immune system.

The morbidity and mortality of major gastrointestinal surgical procedures for cancer (e.g. esophagectomy, gastrectomy, colectomy, hepatectomy and pancreatectomy) demonstrate acceptable rates of complications in elderly patients. The surgical procedure may be tailored to the elderly patient to account for pre-existing disease.

Recent studies investigating the role of endoscopic intervention, such as laparoscopic colectomy for colon cancer, in elderly patients found lower rates of cardiopulmonary-related and overall morbidity than with open colectomy.

Conservation surgery, such as supraglottic laryngectomy and reconstructive subtotal laryngectomy, and conservation surgery of the base of the tongue and hypopharynx and of the breast have shown a moderate mortality rate in elderly patients.

The elderly cancer patient frequently has advanced disease at initial presentation. Recent studies suggest a benefit of palliative surgery in older cancer patients with advanced disease.

Radiotherapy

Little information is available on the practical impact of radiotherapy in elderly cancer patients. Nevertheless, specific trials are underway, mainly in the field of lung cancer treatment. External-beam radiotherapy with conventional fractionation (180–200 cGy/day for 5 days/week) represents the most widely diffused form of treatment in solid tumors in elderly patients. In general, elderly patients are excluded from protocols with unconventional fractionated radiotherapy, due to the fear of increased toxicity, as is sometimes relevant also in younger patients.

Palliative radiotherapy is included in general cancer care of advanced disease. Acute and chronic toxicities of radiotherapy are similar to those shown in younger patients, but subjective tolerance and sometimes compliance are significantly lower than in other age groups.

Chemotherapy

Older patients in overall good health are able to tolerate chemotherapy as well as their younger counterparts, and have similar response rates and time to progression. Although combination chemotherapy is tolerated reasonably well in older patients in good health, a wealth of data suggests that single-agent sequential chemotherapy is associated with similar survival and less toxicity.

Choice of chemotherapeutic regimens is dependent on individual patient characteristics and potentially interacting comorbidities. The development and use of specific regimens for the elderly may produce better outcomes than using an empirically reduced dose of standard regimen.

In phase II or III trials in older patients, the following agents have produced good efficacy and acceptable toxicity:

- non-small cell lung cancer: vinorelbine and gemcitabine
- breast cancer: weekly docetaxel
- bladder cancer: paclitaxel and carboplatin.

Carboplatin is preferable to cisplatin because it causes less renal toxicity and thrombocytopenia and requires a smaller volume of fluid for intravenous administration.

Newer anthracyclines, such as idarubicin and epirubicin, are thought to be less cardiotoxic than traditional anthracyclines and may be useful in older patients. Weekly low-dose epirubicin is tolerated, with negligible toxicity, in women older than 75 years with breast cancer.

The incidence of mucositis can be lowered by using an oral fluoropyrimidine, such as capecitabine, rather than intravenous 5-fluorouracil (5-FU).

Biologically targeted drugs, such as trastuzumab, rituximab and cetuximab, alone or in combination with cytotoxic regimens, can result in effective palliation for many.

The National Comprehensive Cancer Network (NCCN) has issued a set of guidelines for the management of cancer in older individuals:

- a geriatric assessment for all those aged 70 years and older
- adjustment of drug dosage to renal function for those aged 65 years and older
- prophylactic use of granulocyte colony-stimulating factor (G-CSF: filgrastim or pegfilgrastim) for individuals 65 years and older treated with CHOP (cyclophosphamide, doxorubicin, vincristine, prednisone) or chemotherapy of similar dose intensity
- maintenance of hemoglobin levels at 12 g/dl or higher
- preferential use of low-toxicity drugs, such as liposomal doxorubicin, capecitabine, gemcitabine, vinorelbine and weekly taxanes.

Determining the patient- and regimen-specific factors that predict the risk of toxic effects of chemotherapy is clinically relevant. Developing new chemotherapy regimens with similar efficacy but less toxicity for elderly patients should be a priority for future research.

Side effects

Aging is highly individualized, and certain common physiological changes increase the likelihood of toxicity with chemotherapy.

Reduced hematopoietic stem-cell mass and reduced ability to mobilize these cells from the marrow in older persons may slow their recovery after cytotoxic chemotherapy. Similarly, increased destruction of and lower numbers of rapidly renewing mucosal stem cells increase susceptibility to mucositis.

Retrospective analysis of data from clinical trials in patients with solid tumors shows no correlation between age and myelosuppression, the major dose-limiting toxicity of modern chemotherapy regimens. These retrospective studies show that age itself should not be a contraindication for cancer therapy.

Age was found to be a definite independent risk factor for neutropenia in patients older than 60 years with lymphoma in a number of prospective clinical trials of CHOP. These studies found that age is clearly associated with a greater risk of grade 4 neutropenia, neutropenia-related infection and mortality.

The risk of neutropenia and its complications, including death, is highest in the early cycles of chemotherapy. Prophylaxis with a colony-stimulating factor beginning in the first cycle should be considered in elderly patients.

Age was a risk factor for myelosuppression in old women with breast cancer treated with CMF (cyclophosophamide, methotrexate, 5-FU) chemotherapy and patients with lung cancer treated with gemcitabine and vinorelbine. The risk of grade 3 thrombocytopenia and anemia was also higher in old breast cancer patients treated with chemotherapy.

The risk of anthracycline-induced cardiotoxic effects increases with age. Advanced age and reduced glomerular filtration rate appear to be risk factors for peripheral and central neuropathy. Age appears to have no influence on the frequency or severity of nephrotoxicity.

Supportive care

Toxic effects of chemotherapy, such as neutropenia, anemia, mucositis, cardiomyopathy and neuropathy, are more common in elderly patients than in younger patients. This greater susceptibility to the toxicity of chemotherapy may be due, in part, to age-related physiological changes and the higher prevalence of comorbidities in older patients.

Chemotherapy can be made safer by correcting comorbidities and nutritional deficits, but supportive care to ameliorate the side effects of chemotherapy in older patients is needed. It should also be managed in accordance with established guidelines.

Conclusion

The number of elderly patients with cancer will continue to increase. Age-related factors, such as functional and social cognitive impairment, may complicate the management of older patients. The safety, efficacy and convenience of therapy can be optimized with appropriate supportive care interventions. Further studies are needed to assess the activity and toxicity of combined-modality therapy in the elderly as well as to determine specific criteria to select those older patients likely to benefit from treatment.

Further reading

Ayanian JZ, Zaslavsky AM, Fuchs CS et al: Use of adjuvant chemotherapy and radiation therapy for colorectal cancer in a population-based cohort. J Clin Oncol 2003; 21: 1293–1300.

Balducci L, Extermann M: Cancer and aging: an evolving panorama. Hematol Oncol Clin North Am 2000; 14: 1–16.

Balducci L, Extermann M: Management of cancer in the older person: a practical approach. Oncologist 2000; 5: 224–37.

Balducci L, Yates J: General guidelines for the management of older patients with cancer. Oncology (Huntingt) 2000; 14: 221–7.

Balducci L: Geriatric oncology. Crit Rev Oncol Hematol 2003; 46: 211–20.

Balducci L: New paradigms for treating elderly patients with cancer: the Comprehensive Geriatric Assessment and guidelines for supportive care. J Support Oncol 2003; 1(Suppl 2): 30–7.

Coiffier B, Lepage E, Briere J et al: CHOP chemotherapy plus rituximab compared with CHOP alone in elderly patients with diffuse large B-cell lymphoma. N Engl J Med 2002; 346: 235–42.

Extermann M: Measuring comorbidity in older cancer patients. Eur J Cancer 2000; 36: 453–71.

Gridelli C, Maione P, Barletta E: Individualized chemotherapy for elderly patients with nonsmall cell lung cancer. Curr Opin Oncol 2002; 14: 199–203.

Hamerman D: Toward an understanding of frailty. Ann Intern Med 1999, 130: 945–50.

Hurria A, Leung D, Trainor K et al: Factors influencing treatment patterns of breast cancer patients age 75 and older. Crit Rev Oncol Hematol 2003; 46: 121–6.

Lewis JH, Kilgore ML, Goldman DP et al: Participation of patients 65 years of age or older in cancer clinical trials. J Clin Oncol 2003; 21: 1383–9.

Lichtman SM, Villani G: Chemotherapy in the elderly: pharmacologic considerations. Cancer Control 2000; 7: 548–56.

Mahoney T, Kuo YH, Topilow A, Davis JM: Stage III colon cancers: why adjuvant chemotherapy is not offered to elderly patients. Arch Surg 2000; 135: 182–5.

Monfardini S, Balducci L: A Comprehensive Geriatric Assessment (CGA) is necessary for the study and the management of cancer in the elderly. Eur J Cancer 1999; 35: 1771–2.

Morrison VA, Picozzi V, Scott S et al: The impact of age on delivered dose intensity and hospitalizations for febrile neutropenia in patients with intermediate-grade non-Hodgkin's lymphoma receiving initial CHOP chemotherapy: a risk factor analysis. Clin Lymphoma 2001; 2: 47–56.

Popescu RA, Norman A, Ross PJ, Parikh B, Cunningham D: Adjuvant or palliative chemotherapy for colorectal cancer in patients 70 years or older. J Clin Oncol 1999; 17: 2412–18.

Repetto L: Greater risks of chemotherapy toxicity in elderly patients with cancer. J Support Oncol 2003; 1(Suppl 2): 18–24.

Sargent DJ, Goldberg RM, Jacobson SD et al: A pooled analysis of adjuvant chemotherapy for resected colon cancer in elderly patients. N Engl J Med 2001; 345: 1091–7.

Yancik R, Ries LA: Aging and cancer in America: demographic and epidemiologic perspectives. Hematol Oncol Clin North Am 2000; 14: 17-23.

Zachariah B, Balducci L, Venkattaramanabalaji GV et al: Radiotherapy for cancer patients aged 80 and older: a study of effectiveness and side effects. Int J Radiat Oncol Biol Phys 1997; 39: 1125–9.

Care of the imminently dying patient

19

D Tassinari
Infermi Hospital, Italy

M Maltoni
Morgagni–Pierantoni Hospital, Italy

Introduction

End-of-life care is often confused with palliative care, despite the uniqueness of the terminal phase compared with the other stages of cancer. Many authors argue that anticancer treatments and palliative care should be integrated from the start of the natural history of the disease. The terminal stage, however, represents a distinct phase and should be considered as a particular clinical entity within palliative care. While palliative care of advanced and far-advanced disease covers a period of activity of weeks or months, end-of-life **care** is generally limited to a few days or, at most, 1–2 weeks.

Suffering and the terminal phase of the disease

Quality of life should be the primary outcome of palliative care. However, two new topics are becoming increasingly important:

- the quality of death of the patient
- the caregivers and their suffering.

The main difficulties in defining the outcome of supportive care in the final days of life are how to assess the quality of dying, the different components of suffering of the patient and the caregiver, and the relief of patient and caregiver. However, the two dimensions of suffering should not be separated to understand and support the patient and his relatives at the end of life.

Studies have shown that patients and physicians have different opinions of the symptoms influencing the quality of life. Table 19.1 summarizes the five most important symptoms from physicians' and patients' point of view. The differences observed underline once again the difficulties encountered in adopting a correct approach to palliative care. No definitive or validated instruments exist for the assessment of quality of life at the end of life, indicating that close cooperation between physicians and caregivers is

Table 19.1 *The five most important symptoms in the terminal phase of the disease from the physician's (colums 1–3) and patient's (column 4) point of view*

	Hospice	Home care departments	Hospital	Patient's point of view
1	Pain	Fatigue	Pain	Fatigue
2	Anorexia	Pain	Delirium	Drowsiness
3	Intestinal occlusive syndromes	Anorexia	Nausea	Pain
4	Dyspnea	Weight loss	Intestinal occlusive syndromes	Mouth care
5	Fatigue	Dyspnea	Dyspnea	Intestinal occlusive syndromes

fundamental to overcome the intrinsic difficulties inherent in the evaluation of the terminal phase of cancer.

Main symptoms of the terminal phase of the disease

All the clinical symptoms observed during the metastatic phase may also be present in the terminal phase. In six studies on the prevalence of symptoms in patient populations with a survival ranging from 24 hours to 7 days, symptoms were pain (15–99%), dyspnea (17–47%), death rattle (45–56%) and delirium (9–68%). No study has evaluated the prevalence of symptoms due to terminal dehydration.

The physical symptoms present at the end of life require a distinctive approach in management.

Two features are common to all symptoms:

■ A careful distinction must be made between 'difficult' and 'refractory' symptoms in order to facilitate their correct management. For difficult symptoms, control is possible by a combination of specific drugs; for refractory symptoms, a progressive, monitored reduction in the level of patient consciousness is required (palliative sedation: intermittent or continuous, superficial or profound, progressive or sudden).

- Previously used drugs and administration routes undergo progressive simplification. Drugs can be subdivided into the following categories:
  - essential drugs, whose route of administration can be changed (analgesics, antiemetics, sedatives, anxiolytics and anticholinergics)
  - previously essential drugs, which can be stopped (corticosteroids, replacement hormones, hypoglycemics, diuretics, antiarrhythmics and anticonvulsants)
  - drugs that must be discontinued (antihypertensives, antidepressants, laxatives, antiulcer drugs, anticoagulants, antibiotics, iron and vitamins).

Patients with subcutaneous portal systems can receive treatment via their implants.

In all other cases, subcutaneous administration of essential drugs (haloperidol, chlorpromazine, midazolam, lorazepam, metoclopramide, dexamethasone, hyoscine hydrobromide and morphine) via a syringe driver is preferable. Special attention should be paid to potential incompatibilities among the simultaneously infused drugs.

Some analgesics are available in controlled-release formulations for transdermal administration or in immediate-release formulations for sublingual use.

Intractable pain in the terminal phase

Pain represents one of the main burdens for patients with terminal cancer, and opiates are the treatment of choice to control cancer pain. A correct medical approach using the World Health Organization's analgesic ladder and the use of 'opioid rotation' can control about 95% of cancer-related pain syndromes, but a minority of patients experience intractable pain that may require an invasive analgesic approach. 'Refractory' pain benefits from 'palliative sedation'.

End-of-life dyspnea and death rattle

Dyspnea and death rattle are two distressing conditions often occurring at the end of life. The causes of dyspnea in patients with metastatic cancer are related to the stage of the disease, previous and ongoing treatments, and pre-existing or exacerbated nonneoplastic conditions. End-of-life care aims to reduce the distress caused by this symptom, and corticosteroids or central nervous system (CNS) sedatives are the drugs of choice for palliation. The use of sedatives represents one of the more controversial aspects of the palliation of dyspnea in the terminal phase. However, a recent systematic review of literature involving a large number of clinical experiences seems to support their efficacy and safety. The treatment of dyspnea-related distress at the end-of-life should be considered an emergency in palliative care because of the negative impact on the quality of life. Clinicians involved in palliative care should be skilled in the clinical assessment and supportive approach of this symptom.

The death rattle, a fairly distinctive respiration caused by the retention of secretions in the back of the throat, is another symptom frequently present in the dying patient. Patients are unaware of this noise, but family members or caregivers often find it highly disturbing. Reduction of oropharyngeal secretions by anticholinergics and limiting fluid administration are probably the best ways of dealing with this distressing symptom. It must be underlined that oropharyngeal suctioning, often a cause of discomfort, should not be routinely used to resolve the problem, but may be useful in selected patients.

Terminal dehydration

Dehydration represents one of the main problems of patients in the terminal phase, and rehydration remains controversial for ethical and psychological reasons. However, a recent randomized clinical trial showed the benefit of parenteral rehydration for controlling the main symptoms of terminal dehydration in dying cancer patients (Table 19.2).

Delirium and the role of palliative sedation in the terminal phase

The correct management of delirium in the terminal phase of cancer and the identification of patients requiring deep sedation represent two important issues in palliative care. However, there are no definitive data upon which clinical practice guidelines can be based.

Two main problems exist in the clinical approach of the dying patient with delirium: the differential diagnosis between primary and secondary delirium, and the therapeutic approach. Table 19.3 summarizes the main causes of secondary, reversible, delirium, in which an etiological approach would probably be the treatment of choice. However, this type of delirium occurs in almost 50% of previous phases of the disease, and is rare in the terminal phase. In this phase, primary delirium is considered to be a 'physiological' event in the process of death. When conditions favoring secondary delirium can be excluded, the primary approach with sedatives (chlorpromazine, haloperidol or benzodiazepines) is preferred.

Table 19.2 Considerations regarding rehydration in terminally ill cancer patients

Considerations supporting rehydration
• Rehydration would seem to be of benefit in the terminal phase of the disease
• Dehydration may favor terminal delirium or restlessness
• No literature data support the hypothesis that rehydration prolongs the agonic phase of the disease
• Rehydration involves minimal extra care for the team assisting the patient
• Reducing or stopping parenteral rehydration could lead to the suspension of some concomitant palliative treatments
Considerations against rehydration
• Symptoms of the disease are attenuated during the coma that follows dehydration
• Dehydration, in reducing gastrointestinal and bronchial secretions, could also reduce nausea, vomiting and the death rattle
• Dehydration reduces the incidence of ascites and edema
• Parenteral excessive rehydration may worsen the quality of life and of death

Table 19.3 Main causes of secondary delirium

• The addition of new drugs to a pre-existing treatment or modification of the dosage or posology of previously used drugs
• Use of psychoactive drugs (mainly benzodiazepines and antidepressants)
• Acute urinary retention or obstinate constipation or fecaloma
• Discontinuation of chronically used psychoactive drugs
• Dehydration or metabolic abnormalities
• Fever or infections
• Emotive reactions to specific situations or information

There is a great deal of evidence to support the use of palliative sedation in the last part of life, especially for improving the quality of death in a patient with intractable symptoms. At the same time, there is no difference in survival among correctly sedated patients (i.e. in which the objective of sedation is symptom reduction) and nonsedated patients.

Therefore, palliative sedation and euthanasia are completely opposite approaches in terms of intention of treatment, type of procedure and drugs used, and outcome. Palliative sedation is also appropriate for irreversible emergencies in the terminal phase of disease (e.g. acute stridor, massive hemorrhage, myoclonus and convulsions).

Total approach to suffering and quality-of-care assessment

When dealing with the terminal phase of cancer, the responsibility of physicians and caregivers lies in preparing the patient's family for what may still be considered as far-off or uncertain events. They must also learn to use patient-driven coping mechanisms as an indicator of how much the patient wants to know about his/her condition and prognosis. The quality of life of patients and relatives, support for caregivers, and grief support represent the main endpoints of a supportive intervention in end-of-life care. Although no valid instruments exist to evaluate such endpoints, preliminary experiences indicate the need for an assessment of quality of care focused upon patient and caregiver satisfaction in the palliative treatment of advanced or terminal disease. Nevertheless, despite the limits that exist in clinical assessment of the satisfaction of palliative care, an outcome analysis including assessment of quality of life and death in a palliative setting would undoubtedly represent a step forward in improving the clinical approach to total suffering, which is distinctive of the terminal phase of cancer.

Further reading

Bruera E, Sala R, Rico MA et al: Effects of parenteral hydration in terminally ill cancer patients: a preliminary study. J Clin Oncol 2005; 23: 2366–71.

Jennings AL, Davies AN, Higgins JP et al: A systematic review of the use of opioids in the management of dyspnoea. Thorax 2002; 57: 939–44.

Foley KM: Acute and chronic cancer pain syndromes. In: Doyle D, Hanks G, Cherny NI, Calman K (eds), Oxford Textbook of Palliative Medicine, 3rd edn. Oxford: Oxford University Press, 2004: 298–315.

Furst J, Doyle D: The terminal phase. In: Doyle D, Hanks G, Cherny NI, Calman K (eds), Oxford Textbook of Palliative Medicine, 3rd edn. Oxford: Oxford University Press, 2004: 1117–34.

Materstvedt LJ, Clark D, Ellershaw J et al: Euthanasia and physician-assisted suicide: a view from an EAPC Task Force. Palliat Med 2003; 17: 97–101.

Sykes N, Thorns A: The use of opioids and sedatives at the end of life. Lancet Oncol 2003; 4: 312–18.

Communication issues in advanced cancer care

20

PM Parikh
Tata Memorial Hospital, India

SK Shah
Sir H N Hospital and Dr L H Hiranandani Hospital, India

H Malhotra
SMS Medical College, India

GS Bhattacharyya
Apollo Gleneagles Hospital, India

H Khaled
National Cancer Institute, Egypt

> *'DON'T JUST DO SOMETHING, SIT THERE!'*
>
> *Richard Kalish, American social psychologist*

This twist on a well-known line was directed to those whose task involves care for the sick and dying. It is a novel, but pointed, statement that stresses the importance of being really present for people who are suffering, truly hearing their pain, and actually empathizing with them. The issue is not whether 'to communicate or not to communicate', but a question of good versus bad communication. In times of increasing uncertainty, the basic message that patients want to hear is that no matter what, the health-care professionals are going to do all that they can to help them and that they will not be 'abandoned' at any time.

General issues in communication

Communication skills – verbal and nonverbal – are important for oncology health-care providers. Most patients now want to have a better idea of their diagnosis, prognosis, chance of disease recurrence and options in case of treatment failure. Some also have their own preferences about resuscitation or hospice care. Tasks such as information sharing, planning the management of advanced cancers and bereavement care need effective communication, not only with patients but also with their family members. Moreover, the ability to elicit patient preferences and then clearly articulate a plan for treatment is a prerequisite to informed consent.

Oncologists acknowledge that they have had either no or insufficient training in communication skills. Research also suggests that such communication skills do not reliably improve with experience. These factors contribute to additional stress, lack of job satisfaction and emotional burnout among health-care staff.

A prospective study of 130 adults admitted to a hospital with advanced malignancy was conducted to assess how patients perceived information conveyed to them by physicians, as well as the level of communication between patients and health-care staff. This included questions relating to patients' understanding and sense of well-being. Nearly 10% of patients were not even aware of their diagnosis of cancer. Of those who knew their diagnosis, one-quarter stated that the diagnosis was not disclosed in a clear or caring manner, whereas another third of patients had an incomplete understanding of their prognosis. Moreover, patients generally overestimated their understanding of what was actually told to them by hospital medical officers and nurses. The authors concluded that the staff required training in communication skills to handle specifically patients with incurable cancer. They also suggested that professional interpreters should be employed in all instances where the patients and health-care professionals do not share the same mother tongue.

The Study to Understand Prognoses and Preferences for Risks of Treatment (SUPPORT) was a large multicenter study that spanned 5 years. During this time, 4301 patients (seriously ill patients with predicted 50% 6-month mortality rate) were enrolled. It was noted that there was a mismatch between patient preferences and the treatment actually received, obviously due to ineffective communication. Physicians largely ignored or were unaware of the desire of terminally ill patients to be designated as do-not-resuscitate (DNR)/do-not-intubate. The study also found that nurses could not facilitate communication between physicians and patients respecting either physicians' awareness of patients' wishes (about medical care) or the implementation of written DNR orders. The issue is also influenced by physicians' attitudes to life and death and to medical interventions and technology. For instance, physicians' daily work with advanced medical technology may engender a familiarity that makes it difficult for them to comprehend why patients often view ventilators and feeding tubes with anxiety and aversion.

Hence, systematic communication strategies are mandatory. The aim is to:

- facilitate the establishment of a close rapport with the patient
- identify the patient's information preferences
- ensure comprehension of key knowledge and information
- address the patient's emotions in a supportive fashion
- elicit the patient's key concerns
- involve the patient in the treatment plan.

There is an increasing body of evidence that patients want more information from their clinicians than they receive. They also wish to have the opportunity to discuss their preferences and goals of treatment. Objective studies reveal that clinicians spend little time probing the psychosocial aspects of a patient's illness, thereby often failing to make the actual treatment match patient preferences.

Together, the clinician and patient can design a plan of care, acknowledging that the plan is subject to change based on the patient's changing circumstances (e.g. failure to respond to a chosen option in treatment or development of new and disturbing symptoms). At the time of diagnosis, decisions about options in treatment (specific enough to help patients make appropriate plans) should be explored, in a manner that is neither too optimistic nor too pessimistic. Prognostic information should be given in a manner that is truthful in letter and spirit. Subsequent discussion should take into account the patient's concerns, preferences and goals in treatment as well as in life.

The elements necessary to formulate an appropriate care plan include:

- a comprehensive assessment of the medical facts of the individual patient's situation, to include a realistic and accurate appraisal of the likely outcomes
- an understanding of who that person is and what he or she values in life (as well as in death)
- extrinsic factors (e.g. resources and family situation).

Together, these form the assessment backbone for discussing the quality of life that the patient could expect from different therapeutic choices, finally coming to an agreed plan of treatment.

Quill and Brody propose an 'enhanced autonomy' model of decision making in which active dialogue between patient and physician enables the patient to participate in decisions as fully informed of medical realities as possible. They suggest the use of the following 'SPIKES' six-step protocol:

S = get the *S*etting right.
P = understand the patient's *P*erception of the illness.
I = obtain the *I*nvitation to impart information.
K = provide *K*nowledge and education.
E = respond to the patient's *E*motion with empathy.
S = provide *S*ummary strategy.

Nonverbal communicative behaviors of physicians and other health-care professionals also seem to play an important role in meeting the cognitive and affective needs of patients with advanced cancer. Facilitating behaviors such as empathy, touch, comforting gestures and supporting actions are considered essential for humane care.

Communication issues when stopping chemotherapy

For patients with advanced or relapsed cancer, the goals of treatment shift significantly. Treatment is usually directed toward extending life rather than prolonging death, toward reducing suffering (both physical and spiritual), and toward achieving acceptance rather than denial or delusion. Therefore, withholding or withdrawing chemotherapy represents a pivotal time in patient management and requires optimal utilization of communication skills.

Patients do not always hear what physicians tell them. As demonstrated by Weeks et al, patients left on their own tend to be overoptimistic regarding their prognoses. Physicians sometimes withhold the truth from their patients to give them more hope for the future. On the other hand, patients often do not ask questions regarding their illness. The physical and mental stress of a terminal illness can also impede their capacity for understanding, causing otherwise rational people to make irrational choices. This leads to further dissatisfaction with the medical system, causing increased stress, financial strain and risk of malpractice claims. Patients under stress also often transfer the decision-making process either to their physician or to an immediate family member, and neither of them may accurately predict the treatment the patient would have wanted. This situation is even more critical when the health-care professional needs to discuss stopping further cancer-directed systemic therapy (e.g. chemotherapy).

Physicians often feel quite uncomfortable in saying that they cannot effectively fight their patients' cancer, because it might be interpreted as meaning that they have failed. It is much easier simply to give another round of chemotherapy.

Does this mean that clinicians must sit by the bedside, hold patients' hands, and tell them that there is no way to control their cancer? The answer is yes, when that is the truth! The conflict is in deciding how best to communicate this.

Studies indicate that physicians usually rattle off complex information using medical terminology, not realizing exactly how little of this information the patient has actually understood. Weeks and colleagues recommend that to achieve the goals of supporting patient values and minimizing futile therapy, physicians need to change what they tell patients about their prognoses and to be sure that patients understand it. This is the foundation of respect for patient autonomy. The authors state that patients who know their prognosis can make choices about their care that are consistent with their wishes. But this is not enough. Physicians are obligated to initiate patient dialogue, ask what patients want to know, discuss all treatment options (including palliative care) and the likely effect of therapy, and provide estimates of survival. Telling patients the truth about their illness is legally complex. Informed consent also requires that patients be told the risks and benefits of all proposed treatment options, including nontreatment.

It is important to remember that the focus must be on the person rather than the disease. It must be ensured that the patient understands that cure as a treatment goal is no longer realistic, even if that had been a possibility to begin with. In the same conversation, physicians should assure patients that they will not be abandoned, that they will be helped to live for as long as possible and as well as they can.

Strategies that facilitate the transition of care to palliative and comfort measures include:

- reinforcing rapport
- finding out what the patient and family already know
- identifying preferences for receipt of information (amount and complexity)
- giving the information in a sensitive but straightforward manner
- responding to emotions
- redefining the overall goals of treatment given the patient's personal goals, the medical facts and the available technology
- finalizing the care plan, selecting elements based on goals of treatment.

Communication in palliative care

Palliative management should meet the physical, psychological, spiritual and social challenges facing patients and their families, with the objective of enhancing dignity and quality of life.

The key goals of palliative care include:

- optimal pain and symptom control
- psychosocial and spiritual support for the patient and family
- informed decision making
- coordinated services across the continuum of care.

Opportunities to relieve symptoms and achieve meaningful closure to life may be missed when palliative care is considered only after disease-oriented care fails or becomes too burdensome, or when the patient reaches a clearly defined terminal phase. Such an approach only reinforces the negative perception that palliative care means that all else has failed. Patients may also infer incorrectly that relieving symptoms is important only near the end of life. Furthermore, it is sometimes difficult to identify that a particular patient is expected to die in the very near future. Hence, a patient-centered model of care is ideally implemented from the very beginning. This enhances and facilitates a later transition to a palliative approach.

Requirements of a palliative specialist include skills in:

- symptom control
- decision making
- management of treatment complications
- care of the dying
- communication
- psychosocial care
- coordination of care.

Although the techniques of enhancing communication are not unique to the palliative care setting, attention given to communication is heightened when this becomes the primary goal of care. This also requires different communication content. It should incorporate discussion about loss and grief, which may help alleviate psychological distress.

Skills for effective communication in the palliative care setting include:

- listening
- assessment
- facilitation

- techniques for handling difficult questions
- self-awareness.

Additional psychological support can be provided by more open communication regarding end-of-life issues. Patients must cope with significant feelings of fear and loss of their dignity. Additionally, family members may have to cope not only with the cognitive and behavioral changes in their relative, but also with the distress of 'rehearsing' their own future illness if they are genetically at risk. Good communication between patients and their caregivers will provide comfort while discussing loss and impending death, as well as aid in picking up early signs of depression and anxiety.

The focus should therefore be on the barriers that need to be overcome, such as:

- therapeutic 'ennui' (disengagement or difficulty in imagining alternative approaches when active treatment is not available)
- discomfort in discussing end-of-life issues
- belief that symptoms are acceptable or inevitable
- ignorance about palliative care.

Only careful attention to these issues will reinforce the medical team's commitment to ensuring comfort and relief as the illness progresses, and facilitating the seamless, uninterrupted transition from possibility to probability and then inevitability of death.

When palliative care is shared between different locations, good communication is important even among the health-care professionals concerned. They need to keep each other informed of a patient's progress on a real-time basis. Modern technologies, such as electronic summaries and email, are simplifying information sharing. Their widespread use needs to be adopted even more extensively.

Loss of communication due to physical or cognitive changes can be considered a type of 'social death', and families and patients need help to come to terms with the isolation that it causes.

Oncologists and other members of the palliative team are also 'at risk'. Sometimes they fail to communicate with patients or ignore their requests to limit care because of the stress and emotional discomfort occurring when their patients are confronting death. They may be uncomfortable with their own mortality and hence may avoid spending additional time with dying patients. They are also likely to feel themselves failures when they allow a patient to die. This is particularly true when they know that the patient's life could have been prolonged by life support (having been trained to prolong life and overcome disease). In this regard, withholding or withdrawing life-sustaining care can be one of the most difficult actions that a physician has to take.

Breaking 'bad news' is a task often considered daunting. This task is compounded when dealing with death and its meaning. Clinicians may have their own personal fears and sometimes even a death anxiety, which is bound to highlight their lack of training, knowledge and experience in giving bad news. Formal training in communication skills will facilitate implementation and enable optimal utilization of the wide variety of resources available on the subject. Ability to relay difficult information requires physician competence, preparation and time, and the availability of a special facility to communicate in a confidential and private manner.

Death education is not limited to learning only about dying and death. 'Death education' is at the same time 'life education'. Such an education can:

■ help to provide better terminal care during the final stage of life
■ help cancer patients to live the remaining days of their life more fully
■ therefore be helpful in improving their quality of life.

Each of the three involved parties, namely, the medical personnel, the patient, and the family members and friends, can benefit from different aspects of death education.

For patients, it is important to be aware that time is limited and to try to discover the preciousness of what is remaining. Encouraging meditation on the uniqueness of one's own death should be coupled with removal of the taboo on death, making funeral arrangements and considering the possibility of another life after death. They should also complete any unfinished business, be encouraged to take care of personal matters (such as updating their will, and thinking about end-of-life care and advance directives) and discuss these with an appropriate surrogate. They should re-evaluate human relationships and may benefit from life-review therapy.

For the patient's family and friends, it is time to enhance warm communication with the dying patient, and prepare for their own bereavement and grief, as well as use this as an opportunity for personal growth.

Medical personnel should learn to understand the fears and anxieties of a patient facing death. This will help them understand and utilize means to reduce such excessive fears and anxieties. They must also familiarize themselves with the ethical issues related to terminal care. The key is to establish a warm relationship based on trust, which must continue to the end.

Physicians should:

- elicit patient's concerns, goals and values by open-ended questions and following up on the patient's response before discussing specific clinical decisions
- acknowledge patients' emotions, explore their meaning and encourage patients to talk more about difficult topics
- screen for unaddressed spiritual and existential concerns.

As a rule, conversations should be open-minded and nonjudgmental, compassionate and culturally sensitive. Care must be taken not to let personal prejudices and beliefs color this discussion process. A written treatment plan to enhance understanding among all parties is also recommended. This should specifically include decision making about life-sustaining interventions. The preferences and values of patients and their surrogates need to be taken into account. This will also ensure that they are encouraged to become part of the decision-making process. Clinicians must also be prepared to address practical issues in clinical management. These include how to respond to disagreements among staff members and families, the constraints of institutional policies, and misconceptions about the clinical effects and ethics of high-dose narcotics for symptom relief. Such conversations are never easy, because sadness, grief and fear of the unknown are inevitable. Good end-of-life care should help dying patients achieve closure and find meaning in the final phase of their lives.

Communication in the hospice

A hospice serves patients with advanced disease who have accepted that they are dying. Generally, they are expected to live for less than 6 months. A hospice emphasizes multidisciplinary and coordinated care to support patients and their families as they go through the dying process, ideally helping them find peace and acceptance before death. A hospice requires patients to accept a limited prognosis and even 'give up' treatment for their underlying disease.

Hence, the first hurdle is to acknowledge that the patient is likely to die. If the patient (or family) has first confirmed that they want complete information, there is every reason to share the knowledge that the patient is likely to die. This will enhance planning and preparation for death.

Although physicians are reasonably good at predicting who is going to die and when, this is not true of patients. In one study, 82% of patients overestimated their survival, and 59% were decidedly overoptimistic. The choices and consequences of these patients were strikingly different. Those who thought they were going to live for 6 months or more were 2.6 times as likely to choose 'aggressive' anticancer therapy instead of 'palliative' or hospice care. Such patients who received 'aggressive' antineoplastic therapy were 1.6 times more likely to have a hospital readmission, undergo attempted resuscitation, or die while receiving ventilatory support. On the other hand, patients (and families) who accept decisions to move to a residential care facility or hospice may be fraught with guilt, loss and grief.

We must remember that critically ill patients are frequently unable to communicate their wishes. This forces their physicians and family members to make decisions for them – decisions that are of a very personal nature. Patients would want to discuss plans for the end-of-life, but they may need the clinician to initiate the discussion. To protect the right of hospitalized patients, physicians should determine, at a minimum, whether patients wish to be designated as DNR/do-not-intubate and whether patients have provided an advance directive or durable power of attorney for health care. When patients cannot speak (because of intubation, for example), effective communication is still possible (for instance, by nodding and shaking heads). If a physician believes that meaningful communication with a patient is impossible, a surrogate (designated by a durable power of attorney for health care) can speak and decide for the patient.

Communication can also influence ambivalence and uncertainties about power and control in the physician–patient relationship. The physician has gradually taken on a less paternalistic role as more emphasis has been placed on patient autonomy. Educating patients about their diseases and available therapeutic options empowers them to participate more fully in medical decision making and should not be perceived as threatening the physician's authority. As stated earlier, physicians may feel that they, with their greater medical knowledge and experience, are in a better position to make decisions about health care. When faced with difficult decisions about end-of-life care, physicians may even believe that they can relieve the patient's family of guilt, regret and confusion by making tough choices on their own. However, such treatment decisions are not only based on outcome probabilities but may also be influenced by physicians' personal values and priorities. At such times, we need to remember that, as physicians and health-care professionals, we have no right to play God. After all, it is the patient's life that is at stake. The patient's voice must be heard, and the patient's values must be honored.

Additional dilemmas and challenges include:

- issues surrounding accurate determination of prognosis
- concerns about effectively communicating a terminal prognosis while still allowing patients and families to maintain hope
- conflicts of interests for involved clinicians
- potential problems of the current reimbursement mechanisms for hospices (which may be inadequate to meet the needs of all dying cancer patients)
- recognition of diverse cultural needs, and appropriate strategies to meet them.

There are a number of guidelines that health-care workers can use to develop favorable circumstances for the care of terminally ill cancer patients. These include the following:

- The professional interdisciplinary team should be identified and accessible.
- A team leader needs to be designated, and the team should meet to coordinate and review care.
- The team should provide time to listen, understand and analyze what patients and caregivers say and through this ensure that their needs are properly attended to.
- Symptoms should be controlled and reviewed.
- Appropriate domestic, financial, moral and professional support should be provided.
- The patient and domestic caregiver should feel involved in care and management. They should aware of the help that is available as well as how to help themselves.
- The team should ensure delivery of care for the terminal stages and bereavement according to the plan mutually agreed upon (home visits, evening services and 24-hour availability of medical assistance in emergencies).

Additional recommendations for improving family-centered palliative care are as follows:

- Determine key family members (as identified or agreed to by the patient) and include them in the documented multidisciplinary care plan.
- Prepare family members for roles associated with supporting a dying relative.
- Provide written information to supplement verbal guidance in a structured manner.
- Assist family members with skills to optimize patient comfort.

- Regularly assess individual family caregiver needs for respite, information and support.
- Assess the need for spiritual and bereavement support prior to the patient's death.

Spiritual well-being offers some protection against end-of-life despair. Breitbart et al noted that the desire for hastened death among terminally ill cancer patients is not uncommon, with depression and hopelessness being their strongest indicators. They suggested that interventions addressing depression, hopelessness and social support appear to be important aspects of adequate palliative care.

When a person chooses to die at home, the family also needs to be specifically briefed about:

- the treatment outline for pain and symptom control (when to identify suboptimal control)
- the role of each health-care team member (who to call for help and when)
- aids and equipment (which ones will help at home and when)
- the actual dying process (explaining to the family how death usually occurs) and potentially distressing events (expected and unexpected, such as terminal confusion, vomiting or hemorrhage)
- what to do at the time of and immediately after death (funeral arrangements and death certificates).

Communication issues in patients' families

Often, families 'cascade through an avalanche' of emotional upheavals while patients are struggling with the sequelae of their illness. We all agree that there is no substitute for talking to the patient. Similarly, the family, particularly the patient's surrogate, should also be included as a key player requiring attention in the overall communication plan.

Family caregivers play a central role in the well-being of most patients. It is therefore important that attention be given to their needs and experiences. However, this happens only rarely. Caregivers' needs are usually overshadowed by concerns about the patient's comfort, practical care, information needs and emotional support. It is clear that optimal care cannot be provided unless the physician adopts a family-oriented approach. Such an approach usually requires only a little additional time or effort. However, it profoundly affects the ability of the patient and family to cope with the illness. Physicians should routinely gather data about the patient's family system and use it in understanding the unique issues that the patient is likely to face in adapting to the illness. The physician's goal should be to anticipate how it will affect the family at its current stage of the life cycle. The physician should also recognize how the patient's family, in turn, is currently affecting the patient's experience of the illness.

If the patient's loved ones must make life-and-death decisions on the patient's behalf, they will probably have feelings of grief, guilt and confusion. Truth about prognosis might have a significant effect on family members required to make decisions on behalf of patients with terminal cancer. Relatives should not feel 'left out' or 'in the way' at a crucial time when impending death is having a profound impact. A lack of sensitivity among doctors and staff can affect the grieving process adversely.

Just as many professionals feel uncomfortable in talking about the end of life, family members face similar challenges in expressing their feelings and asking questions about the patient's prognosis. Caring physicians can greatly ease such burden at times of crisis by:

- understanding the need for relatives to be with the terminally ill patient
- being available for help and comfort of the patient
- designating a team member to be informed of the patient's condition and of impending death
- facilitating expression of emotions among family members and comforting them
- answering the family's questions honestly and in simple terms
- providing reassurance that the best possible care is being given.

The primary family caregivers at home also need to be appraised of the disruption that is likely to occur in their life. Patients will be able to do or decide less and less. Hence, family caregivers will have to take on a role that evolves in tune with the patient's deterioration. They will have to take care of and protect the patient, be their emotional counselor and family spokesperson, and look after unfinished legal and other family matters. It is no wonder that caregivers admit that the terminal phase is the most exhaustive time of their life.

After a patient dies, clinicians should be familiar with generally recognized patterns of behavior that are indicative of a normal mourning process. This knowledge may help clinicians recommend the intervention of other professionals (either medical or pastoral) in a timely manner.

Collusion needs special attention. It implies that information (about diagnosis, prognosis and medical details about the moribund person) will be withheld by some persons and not shared with significant others. It also means that appropriate and complete medical information is not disclosed to either the patient or other relatives. It is a universal phenomenon and is often unnoticed in many families. It is of two types:

- the medical team colluding with relatives such that the patient is 'in the dark' (a more common situation)
- the doctors colluding with the patient and not informing the spouse and other family members and relatives about the patient's illness.

Collusion can lead to poor communication between health-care professionals, the patient and family members. In such a situation, it is important to explore the reasons for such collusion and examine the patient–family members relationship(s). This will guide the path to break collusion so as to resolve the underlying issues. The presence of collusion can lead to psychological problems in the patient and, later, problems with grief in relatives. When the family members want the health-care team not to discuss details with the patient, it is important to prevent or resolve such collusion by going through the following steps:

- Elicit the reasons for withholding information from the patient.
- Counsel about the harm of such a collusion.
- Seek approval to confirm the validity of their reasons with the patient.
- Check the level of awareness in the patient.
- Give feedback to family members about the patient's level of awareness or readiness to know about the disease.
- Encourage conversation between the patient and family members.
- Provide any clarification or answers to doubts.
- Counsel regarding any guilt or unpleasant emotions among the concerned parties.

Conclusion

Effective communication is an important and often neglected aspect in optimal patient management. This is even more so for patients with advanced cancer or those who are terminally ill. The need for formal training in communication skills has been recognized only recently, even though validated resource material is already available. A multidisciplinary team approach will ensure that communication is improved with patients and their family members. This will enable proper identification of unmet needs and areas of conflict. It will also help the health-care team to set goals and schedule treatment plans that are in keeping with the patient's desire, the family's circumstances and their ethnic/cultural requirements. Such a scheme will also ensure that the family has an opportunity to share in the decision-making process, remain satisfied with the delivery of care, and not have an undue burden of guilt or abnormal mourning. Channels for effective communication therefore need to be set up early in the illness and to be strengthened as the patient moves from palliation to treatment for the terminally ill.

Further reading

Chan A, Woodruff RK: Communicating with patients with advanced cancer. J Palliat Care 1997; 13: 29–33.

Chen H, Haley WE, Robinson BE, Schonwetter RS. Decisions for hospice care in patients with advanced cancer. J Am Geriat Soc 2003; 51: 789–97.

Christakis NA, Asch DA: Physician characteristics associated with decisions to withdraw life support. Am J Public Health 1995; 85: 367–72.

Griffin JP, Nelson JE, Koch KA et al: End-of-life care in patients with lung cancer. Chest 2003; 123(1 Suppl): 312S–31S.

Hudson P: Palliative care. Home-based support for palliative care families: challenges and recommendations. Med J Aust 2003; 179 (Suppl 6): S35–S7.

Nelson CJ, Rosenfeld B, Breibart W et al: Spirituality, religion, and depression in the terminally ill. Psychosomatics 2002; 43: 213–20.

Quill TE, Brody H: Physician recommendations and patient autonomy: finding a balance between physician power and patient choice. Ann Intern Med 1996; 125: 763–9.

Smith T, Swisher K: Telling the truth about terminal cancer. JAMA 1998; 279: 1746–8.

SUPPORT Principal Investigators: A controlled trial to improve care for seriously ill hospitalized patients. The Study to Understand Prognoses and Preferences for Outcomes and Risks of Treatments (SUPPORT). JAMA 1995; 274: 1591–8.

Weeks JC, Cook EF, O'Day SJ et al: Relationship between cancer patients' predictions of prognosis and their treatment preferences. JAMA 1998; 279: 1709–14.

21 Self-care

E Maex
ZNA Middelheim, Belgium

C De Valck
Limburgs Universitair Centrum, Belgium

Introduction

People working in a radiology or radiotherapy ward carry a small device that is adjusted regularly and serves to detect accidental radiation. Radiation is seen as a risk factor, and an accidental overdose is a potential hazard. In the case of a positive result, protective and preventive measures can be taken. This is standard procedure.

Caregivers working in oncology are often not aware of the continuous 'emotional radiation' to which they are exposed. Despite a gigantic amount of research on stress, frequent emotional contacts and burnout, the emotional side of being an oncologist is often ignored as a risk factor and potential health hazard.

Burnout

In recent years, burnout in medical professions has drawn a lot of attention. The phenomenon has been studied and reported by the European Medical Association, and it was found that burnout can be a threat to the quality of medical care.

Burnout is characterized by physical and psychological exhaustion that is no longer compensated by rest, loss of concentration, denial of emotions, reduction of the medical relation to strictly scientific aspects of the disease, loss of empathy, and cynicism as a defense mechanism.

In the literature, the prevalence of burnout in physicians is 30–60%. Oncologists are among those most at risk. The Maslach Burnout Inventory, a self-reporting instrument, may be used to measure burnout.

Studies focusing on the relation between burnout and patient care showed that doctors with symptoms of burnout communicated less well with their patients. Treatment was poorly discussed and explained, and questions from the patient were left unanswered more often than by doctors without symptoms of burnout.

This shows the importance of self-care for patient care and the importance of burnout prevention.

A model of self-care

Coping may be categorized as problem-oriented and emotion-oriented coping.

Problem-oriented coping is the usual coping mechanism by health-care professionals, and most are experienced in this coping technique.

Emotional coping is more difficult. It is important that health-care professionals can recognize emotional stress by a personal 'emotional dosimeter' and can apply a model of self-care.

Detection

Basically, the only personal stress detector is one's own body, since it is the only instrument that enables feelings. To keep track of the stress to which we are exposed, we need to keep track of the body. Figure 21.1 shows an 'emotional dosimeter'. It is based on two questions about the actual experience:

- How much energy does one have (x-axis)?
- How much tension does one experience (y-axis)?

This can be rated by a visual analogue scale (VAS).

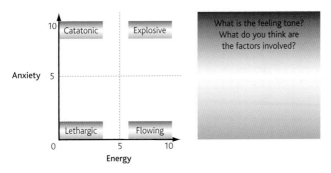

Figure 21.1 *Emotional dosimeter for detection of emotional stress*

The combined result places one at an actual moment in a square marked by four theoretical extremes:

- Low energy–low tension would be a state of lethargy more dead than alive.
- Low energy–high tension would be a catatonic state, in which someone remains unmoved, due to lack of energy, while the tension mounts to the unbearable.
- High energy–high tension adds energy to the previous state, bringing about a highly explosive situation fueled by high anxiety and energy.
- High energy–low tension is what is sometimes called 'the flow', an effortless state unhampered by anxiety tension or fatigue.

Obviously, a state of low tension and high energy (flowing) is what we most aspire to. However, these extremes in themselves rarely occur. They merely serve as a guideline.

Next to the diagram are two questions.

1. 'What is the feeling tone?' Next to bodily tension and energy, there is an emotional value to feelings. This can be sadness, joy, anger or any other of the large range of human emotional experiences.

2. 'What do you think are the factors involved?' We may not always be aware of what brings about bodily and emotional states, but this question invites us to reflect on what is going on.

Taking care

As noted, we are not always, not to say rarely, in this state of low tension and high energy (flowing). When we realize that our bodily and emotional state is not going well, we need to take care.

In taking care of difficult emotions, human beings have basically two possible strategies. We can choose to distract ourselves from the emotion, putting our thoughts on something else, or we can allow them in. Both strategies make sense. It is all about balance. Sometimes, people, unable to distract themselves, get lost in their feelings and fail to notice what else life has to offer. Some people, on the other hand, lose all their energy in running away from their feelings, but, despite that, they are constantly taken over by them. Time is healing, but only if we take time for what is going on emotionally and allow emotions to be taken into account.

Both strategies can be practiced alone or with others. This gives the four quadrants shown in Figure 21.2.

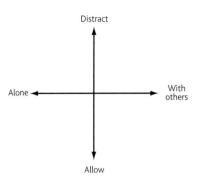

Figure 21.2 *Coping mechanisms*

When we feels sad, we can put on some joyful music to lighten our mood (*distracting–alone*). But we can also opt for a sad song and allow the feeling in (*allowing–alone*). Given the large number of songs about lost loves, there seems to be a market for this.

We do not have to be alone with our feelings. We can share them with close friends or with colleagues when they are work-related (*allowing–with others*). We can also have great fun with friends or colleagues and discuss everything but our sadness (*distracting–with others*).

None of these strategies is in itself better than others. Comfort in dealing with difficult emotions is a function of how freely we can move through the four quadrants. It is a useful exercise to draw the diagram on a piece of paper, and fill in the four quadrants to identify what strategies one personally has at hand when in an unpleasant emotional state. What strategies are lacking or could be cultivated more?

Further reading

Maslach C, Jackson SE: MBI: Maslach Burnout Inventory: Manual Research and Edition. University of California. Palo Alto, CA: Consulting Psychologists Press, 1986.

Shanafelt TD, Bradley KA, Wipf JE, Back, AL: Burnout and self reported patient care in an internal medicine residency program. Ann Intern Med 2002; 136: 358–67.

22 Psycho-oncology in palliative care

R Mathys
ZNA Middelheim, Belgium

Introduction

Until the 1950s, the scientific community paid little attention to psychosocial issues in cancer patients. This was partly because many scientists felt sure that, by the end of the century, the battle against cancer would have been won. Every effort was put into basic and clinical research. The focus of interest was the tumor and, to a lesser extent, the patient. Surgery, radiotherapy and medical oncology became the three pillars on which cancer treatment was based. Diverse concomitant societal and medical developments made psychosocial oncology the fourth pillar of cancer treatment.

Development of psycho-oncology

- There was a renewed interest in the body–mind relationship as described by psychosomatic medicine. The awareness of the complexity of the interaction of body and mind gave birth to the field of psychoneuroimmunology. Spiegel stressed the need to take the mind–body interaction seriously in the design of any health-care program, since poorly adapted patients may have a worse prognosis.
- The doctor–patient relationship, which is the cornerstone of the art of medcine, underwent a drastic change: from the vertically parternalistic relationship to a horizontal relationship in which doctor and patient are equally important but have different expertise. The physician acts as the expert in medical matters, while the patient is the only expert on his or her quality of life. The doctor discusses different options with the patient, and they decide together how to proceed: the relationship has developed to a partnership.
- Palliative care developed in response to the need in care of dying patients and their family. Saunders introduced the concept of total pain with physical, psychological, social and spiritual dimensions.

- Razavi and others showed that communication between patients, their families and professional caregivers could be improved by training, and that teamwork had a positive impact on the quality of life of the patient. Patients who are satisfied with the doctor–patient interaction understand more about their illness and the complexity of treatment and medication use. They are more compliant with instructions and treatment plans. They demonstrate better psychological adjustment and are less anxious and depressed. These patients are generally more satisfied with their care and their professional caregivers.
- The development of psychotropic drugs in the 1950s enabled the treatment of insomnia, fear and depression. These drugs were a valuable help to psychological support.
- Customer and self-help groups also played an important role in the development of psychosocial oncology.

Psycho-oncology and palliative care

Psycho-oncology addresses the psychological, social and behavioral dimensions of cancer from two perspectives:

- the psychological responses of patients and their families at all stages of cancer
- the influence on morbidity and mortality.

In palliative care, two factors are important in the field of psycho-oncology:

- The development of new treatments and better supportive care made cancer a chronic disease. Although patients might not be cured, they may live for a longer time. The drawback is that patients are confronted with persistent side effects, constant interference with quality of life, stressful uncertainty of the future and fear of death. The challenge for these patients is how to live well while being ill. The period from diagnosis till death (Figure 22.1) may be very short – a few weeks or months but may extend over years. Palliative oncology and palliative care have to be integrated from the start of diagnosis: patients should know that the switch from cure to care is not the end of their life. Good palliative care is prepared by good psychosocial care during the chronic phase of the disease. This is reflected by the concept of continuing care.
- The phase of palliative care is characterized by a complex interaction of physical and psychological problems. Palliative care patients have, on average, 8–12 different symptoms. Some of these problems may be clustered as chronic pain, depression, fatigue, memory and concentration

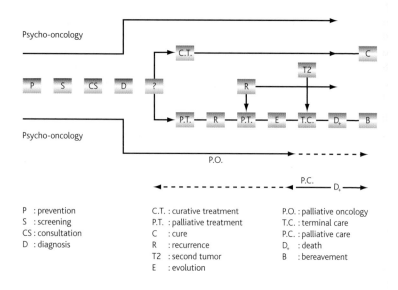

P : prevention
S : screening
CS : consultation
D : diagnosis

C.T. : curative treatment
P.T. : palliative treatment
C : cure
R : recurrence
T2 : second tumor
E : evolution

P.O. : palliative oncology
T.C. : terminal care
P.C. : palliative care
D⁺ : death
B : bereavement

Figure 22.1 Hallmarks of psychosocial oncology

problems, and insomnia. Most physicians are qualified to recognize and treat complex physical problems (e.g. pain, nausea and vomiting, fatigue), but are less trained to recognize the psychological and social needs of palliative care patients.

The American Society for Psychosocial and Behavioral Oncology and AIDS (ASPBOA) opted for the word 'distress' to describe the problems of cancer patients and their families, to avoid stigmatization of psychosocial problems. This term was chosen because it recognized that distress is a response to cancer characterized by sadness, worry and fears, and that it may increase and reach a level that requires intervention.

When dealing with psychosocial problems, it is important to realize that the vast majority of patients do not have a pre-existent psychiatric disorder, but that the distress is directly related to the cancer and its treatment. The Psychosocial Collaborative Oncology Group determined the prevalence of psychiatric disorders in 215 cancer patients, who were ambulatory or hospitalized with a wide range of cancer type and stage in three cancer centers, by the DSM-III classification. About half (53%) of the patients adjusted normally to the stress due to cancer without a diagnosable psychiatric disorder; 47% had a clinically apparent psychiatric disorder, of whom 68% showed reactive anxiety and depression (adjustment disorders with depressed or anxious mood); 13% had major depression; and 8% had an organic mental disorder (delirium). On average, 25% of all cancer patients experience severe depressive symptoms in the course of their disease.

It is mandatory to recognize distress promptly, since physical and psychological symptoms often influence each other and have a negative impact on the quality of life. Cancer patients with advanced disease are a particularly vulnerable group, since it is known that the incidence of pain, depression and delirium increases with physical debilitation and advanced illness.

ASPBOA pleads for greater awareness of the underrecognition and the need to manage distress and psychological problems in cancer and maintain standards of care.

When patients are confronted with the end of their life, providing psychosocial care is challenging. Often it goes beyond the capacity of the individual caregiver and needs an intelligent, interdisciplinary team approach. The assessment of psychosocial need may be difficult, since people are reluctant to admit that they are losing grip on their life.

Conclusion

Psychosocial interventions may help patients and their families cope with cancer at all stages and its treatment. The old biomedical concept of disease should yield to a global, biopsychosocial approach.

The main skill that oncologists need to develop is the total management of the patient with cancer, and patients confronted by the end of their life should be offered psychosocial care. This care should be integrated in the context of the patient's own culture and should be provided by a team of professional caregivers, since it may go beyond the capacities of the individual caregiver. It needs intelligent, interdisciplinary teamwork.

The assessment of psychosocial needs may be hampered by the fact that people are reluctant to lose grip on their life. Therefore, oncologists should rely on their psychosocially trained team members.

Further reading

O'Neill B, Fallon M. ABC of palliative care. Principles of palliative care and pain control. BMJ 1997; 315: 801–4.

Razavi D, Delvaux N, Hopwood P. Improving communication with cancer patients. A challenge for physicians. Ann NY Acad Sci 1997; 809: 350–60.

Spiegel D, Bloom JR, Kraemer H, Gottheil E: Effect on psychosocial treatment on survival of patients with metastatic breast cancer. Lancet 1989; ii: 888–91

Bereavement

RM Smeding
Institute for Educational Expertise in Palliative and
Bereavement Care, Germany

Introduction

After death, normal grieving may last from 10 days (exceptional) to 4 years or longer. Normal grieving may present physical, emotional, social, intellectual and spiritual issues, and depends on a person's living experience. Recent longitudinal research suggests that Freud's suggestion of 'cutting all ties that bind' is done by only one-third of the bereaved, be they bereaved spouses or parents.

Closure of an actively grieving period varies between integration by a continued, but altered, presence of the deceased, a ritualized attendance to particular dates (e.g. birthdays) or total closure.

Current research identifies bereavement difficulties for some 20% as unhelpful avoidance, lack of basic life skills (emotional or problem-solving-oriented, or both) or chronic grief.

Psychotherapeutic interventions may be needed and may be enhanced by complementary social learning via bereavement support groups.

Cancer-related personal experiences may trigger dormant or presumably finalized grief processes.

Etiology

Kübler-Ross's five stages of grief, before or after death, derive from early historical developments in bereavement care. Grief patterns are related to:

- developmental stage
- relationship to deceased
- pattern of bonding
- life-span issues (e.g. early married with small children)
- circumstances surrounding death.

Causal research currently focuses on attachment patterns, and meaning and stress theories.

Assessment

Active grief may cause:

- physical complaints (muscle pains, nausea, lack of appetite or tachycardia)
- memory loss, apathy or confused states
- emotional instability or depression-like symptoms
- desire to die 'toward deceased' (differential diagnosis with suicidal intentions should be assessed by a psychiatrist or psychotherapist!)
- a strong need to find meaning.

The person may be at different stages of the grief trajectory according to age, personality, relationship to deceased, or working circumstances.

There may be a direct relationship between a patient's unmet psychological needs and the development of bereavement difficulties for the partner.

Doctors might help to prevent pathological grief by identifying the following risk factors:

- manifest depression
- strong aggression
- denial behavior
    - denial of regression of illness
    - flight into work
- overprotective behavior
    - of self (including abandonment before death)
    - of others (e.g. exclusion of children).

Complicated or pathological grief

Complicated or pathological grief is a syndrome that requires the co-occurrence of a series of symptoms. It is usually not diagnosed before 2 months after death, with the exception of survivors posing a direct threat to themself or to their surroundings, or when death has not been 'recognized' by the partner, in which case immediate intervention may prevent further harm.

Treatment

Provision of care covers the period of dying, death and bereavement. Cancer and its effects may trigger new or existing patterns of difficult communication, coping or avoidance. Doctors are considered to play important roles in support and helpful relationship. Active modeling of adequate behavior requires caring and realistic communication, free from the use of *jargon* (e.g. professional expressions or abbreviated referrals).

Grieving persons and their relationships require psycho-oncological consultation and, if necessary, treatment.

Preparing for death and loss

When death is imminent, medical caregivers and their team should take an inventory of the relationships and situation. This may be done before but at the latest during the terminal phase. The factors to be determined are as follows:

- who holds key leadership in the system of relationships
- who will take this loss especially hard
- additional burdens to future grief
- family/relationship network and resources.

'Preparedness for a loved one's death' and 'having said goodbye' are influential factors for healthy grief trajectories.

At death: 180-seconds treatment

At death, the surviving relationship system usually needs professional attention. A doctor's care can contribute to the prevention of loss-induced symptoms by giving time and attention after the patient's death (so-called 180 seconds treatment). Caregivers' behavior at those moments may have a lifelong influence.

Helpful behavior at the time of death may include:

- extending sympathy over the loss of family member/partner, surpassing empty phraseology
- expressing the importance of informal caregivers' contributions to patient care
- inclusion of those who 'haven't made it to the moment of death'
- indication of availability for 'visit-after-death'. A discussion of 'leftover' medically based questions alleviates or dispels myths as to end-of-life medical care, the story of which is now going into the survivor's biography and, repeatedly told, into the community (e.g. hydration issues, withdrawal of food or change of medication).

Systems found to be 'at risk' for future complicated grief require postponement of case closure at death. Scheduling psychosocial/pastoral consultation(s) after death allows the original health-care system involved in a patient's illness and death to use its expertise, aimed at early prevention of pathological grief. As the impact of the loss unfolds, further care by assessments and/or referrals is facilitated.

Precautions

1. Adequate coping before or at the time of death, if combined with risk factors, should invoke care to be extended beyond these moments.
2. Normal losses (e.g. losing one's parent at an advanced age) can still trigger strong grief, including confusion, anger or lack of appetite. Symptoms can remain present for months, without being pathological.
3. Elderly people, especially, accumulate loss (with peers and friends dying), which aggravates new bereavement when their partner or child dies.
4. It is a myth that children do not realize loss. At any moment of the illness and the subsequent loss trajectory, involving children by way of adequate communication and care, respecting age and development, has been shown to be helpful.
5. History taking should therefore always include assessment of the patient and system as to current losses, covering at least the last 18 months.

Further reading

Christ, GH: Healing Children's Grief; Surviving a Parent's Death from Cancer. New York: Oxford University Press, 2000.

Kübler-Ross E: On Death and Dying . New York: Scribner, 1997.

Lichtenthal WG, Cruess DG, Prigerson HG: A case for establishing complicated grief as a distinct mental disorder in DSM-V. Clin Psychol Rev 2004; 24: 637–62.

Monroe B, Kraus F: Brief Interventions with Bereaved Children. Oxford: Oxford University Press, 2005.

Neimeyer RA: Meaning Reconstruction and the Experience of Loss. Washington, DC: American Psychology Association, 2000.

Stroebe M, Hanson R, Stroebe W, Schut H (eds), Handbook of Bereavement Research: Consequences, Coping and Care. Washington, DC: American Psychology Association, 2001.

Existential and spiritual issues

ND de Stoutz
Forch, Switzerland

Prevalence and definitions
Existential issues

At a crossroads in a person's life, existential questions arise. Patients cannot acknowledge the diagnosis of cancer without having at least a fleeting thought about the possibility of their death. Therefore, the prevalence of existential issues in cases of advanced cancer is to be assumed to be 100%.

Spirituality

Spirituality is considered to be the vehicle through which persons encounter the mysteries of their own life and death, and their calling to be members of their family, their community and the cosmos. Paradoxically, the journey into death is sometimes considered to be the ultimate vehicle for spiritual discovery. Important elements of a model of spirituality are the following:

- becoming (values, self-esteem and creativity)
- belonging (relationships, community and culture)
- finding meaning (journey, mortality, suffering and hope)
- transcending (awe and wonder, nature, God or Gods, the afterlife).

Spiritual issues

'The search for meaning is a basic human need' (V Frankl). It seems wise to assume that 100% of patients with advanced cancer have some form of spiritual issues.

Total pain is a distress with physical, emotional, social, bureaucratic, financial and spiritual components (C Saunders).

Religion

In a general sense, religion means the search for or the offer of a connection to a 'great transcendence'; of a way from the finite to the infinite, from self to the totally different.

Religions have their system of symbols, which imply and explain each other; these are meditated in individual contemplation and common celebrations, and/or enacted in rituals. This provides a framework for the individual believer's spirituality, which is recognized diversely by different religious traditions.

Believers are not only comforted but also challenged by their religion.

Nonreligious spirituality

Up to 30% of patients in Western countries deny religious affiliation. Yet 95% of people claim to believe in a deity. Many with or without a religion tend to 'help themselves' in a variety of religions without having an organized belief system. They all have an underlying spirituality, which is based on the yearning for meaning, shared by all humans.

Signpost

'Hope is not optimism, not the confidence that an outcome will be good. It is the certainty that things have a meaning, whatever the outcome.' (V Havel).

Etiology

'Physiopathology'

Signals from the deep, spiritual level of experience may influence the physical, psychological and relational state. They can increase distress, manifesting as a variety of medically unspecific problems. On the other hand, tapping into the resources of spirituality can be an invaluable help in coping.

Spiritual issues

Causes of existential or spiritual issues are largely irrelevant, while their effect on the patient's suffering must trigger adequate responses by the health-care team.

The dimensions of spirituality, as described by many authors, are experienced in a variety of ways along a continuum from the most helpful to the most distressing (Table 24.1).

Table 24.1 Helpful and distressing extremes in dimensions of spirituality

Spiritual dimensions (as listed by PW Pruyser)	Distressing extreme	Helpful extreme
Awareness of the Holy (sense of reverence, awe)	Punitive deity, fear of judgment	Contemplation, meditation, worship
Acceptance of benevolence of the divine	Immature bargaining, striving for power/influence over the divine	Trust to be helped, gratitude
Being responsible, repentent	Unresolved experiences, resentments	Self-acceptance, including one's dark sides; interest in becoming a better person
Faith (being open and committed)	Impossibly demanding standards, confusion, doubts	Capacity to enjoy, curiosity to let oneself be surprised/changed
Sense of providence	Fear of abandonment	Courageously and confidently facing the future
Involvement	Doubt of efficacy of spiritual practices, feeling of being a burden	Creativity; doing things for loved ones, carers, community

Spiritual needs

Spiritual needs are those for meaning, purpose, fulfillment, connectedness, love, forgiveness, forgiving, reconciliation, truth, hope and transcendence.

Whether a patient is sailing on calm waters or fighting his way through a storm or across a desert, needs do exist that he may or may not be able to provide for on his own! Unmet spiritual needs cause clinical manifestations such as:

■ uncontrollable pain or other physical symptoms
■ anxiety, sadness and depression, direct statements of despair, hopelessness, suicidal ideation and request for euthanasia
■ manipulative behavior, irritability, anger and agressiveness.

Signpost

Healing is the process of becoming whole, as opposed to being cured. The word 'wholesome' is used in this chapter for anything that contributes to healing.

Assessment
Awareness

Intuition is a 'diagnostic tool' that should be developed as carefully as any other clinical skill. To do this, physicians need to be aware of their own spirituality and possibly find ways to regenerate their energy through it. This opens their receptiveness and helps to pick up the metaphors that allow a glimpse into a patient's spirituality.

Formal assessment

Several assessment instruments are proposed in the literature. For a first assessment, those making no specific reference to formal religious practice are the most useful, as they allow the patient to decide whether or not to use religious language.

The shortest questionnaires can be integrated into medical history taking, but other members of a multidisciplinary team may use more detailed instruments.

Several acronyms have been proposed, which stand for questions to be asked. This needs to be done in a way that is sensitive and open enough to accommodate any sort of belief system. The exact wording should be what each physician feels comfortable with.

FICA (after C Puchalski)

F – Faith: What do you believe in that gives meaning to your life?

I – Importance: What influence does this have on how you take care of yourself?

C – Community: Is this of support to you? How? Do you share this with a group of people?

A – Address: How would you like me/your health-care providers to address these issues in your care?

SPIRIT (after TA Maugen)

S – spiritual belief system

P – personal spirituality

I – integration with a spiritual community

R – ritualized practices and restrictions

I – implications for medical care

T – terminal events planning.

Ongoing assessment

Repeating part or all of the assessment may be indicated in some situations. Listening to the patient, observing nonverbal language and asking questions are part of good clinical practice.

Audit

When one audits spiritual care, it is important to keep in mind that an apparent deterioration in 'spiritual status' can well be an appropriate stage in a patient's spiritual journey.

Signpost

Did you notice that this chapter is full of metaphors of journeying?

General intervention options

The goal of spiritual interventions is to increase opportunities for reconciliation and healing, by:

- **supporting** wholesome spirituality
- **helping** patients with distressing spiritual issues to shift their focus and **access spiritual resources**.

The approach to existential and spiritual issues needs to be interdisciplinary, and physicians can do more than just delegating. If the physician–patient relationship allows an approach to such topics very naturally, the physician can go along with the patient for a few steps or offer interventions as listed below.

Minimal contribution of physicians

■ During first interviews, repeatedly expressing understanding and solidarity provides a basis for a trusting person-to-person relationship. After that, be true to your word!

■ Be yourself, allow your vulnerability to show as well as your confidence.

■ **Excellent symptom control opens space for the patient to attend to spiritual matters!**

■ Do a spiritual assessment. That in itself triggers reflection and a search for meaning. Accept discussion of issues if patients want to expand.

■ Refer to a chaplain, for therapies and other help if appropriate and acceptable.

Join team effort

■ In recognizing the metaphors that a patient uses. The relevance of a metaphor can be tested by repeating it or taking it half a step further, allowing the patient to expand and explain without feeling stupid, or to retreat and claim respect for his or her inner secret.

■ In creating an environment that allows for spirituality to be lived (e.g. tranquility or beauty).

■ In respecting other team members' contributions to spiritual care.

■ In encouraging and showing interest in a patient's spiritual journey.

■ If necessary, in proposing activities (Table 24.2) or therapies that may help the patient.

Signpost

Questions such as 'Why me?' are important to acknowledge, but it is important not to answer them and stifle the exploration of the suffering. The response should open a process that may help the patient.

Religious intervention options

In most instances, the goal of religious intervention is to put the **merciful aspects** of the patient's religion into perspective. Religious observances also need to be respected, and accommodated in health-care institutions.

Table 24.2 *Examples of activities helping patients to attend to their spiritual needs*

Therapies that can help the patient become whole	
Relaxation, dance, massage:	Reconciliation with own body
Art therapy :	Symbolic life review, creativity, beauty
Guided imagery:	A safe way to explore the deep level of experience

Assessment

An individual's spirituality can be expressed within the framework provided by an organized religion or denomination, yet it will be unique for each individual, as it is shaped and influenced by life experience, culture and other personal factors.

Migrants tend to become more attached to their religion than they might have been while in their own country. Patients and families from politically unstable countries may not wish to have contacts with a religious leader, for fear of repression or persecution. Discuss it with them before arranging visits from anyone representing their religious community!

The needs of each patient have to be assessed individually through direct questions.

Care

In caring for religious patients, the crucial factor is not the theological content of their religion but the experience of having their beliefs taken seriously. Patients and their families can have differing or even conflicting views. Mutual respect needs to be encouraged, but distress on both sides is not always avoidable and has to be dealt with, the goal being acceptance and reconciliation, not conversion.

In many hospitals, chaplaincy or nursing staff will have information available on the most important religions, including contact addresses of religious communities.

Although Table 24.3 cannot give a full account of all tenets of all religions, it may be of help to accommodate the religious needs of patients in an institutional context.

In many cultures and religions, grief is shown openly: loud wailing and motor reactions may seem exaggerated, and may be shocking for other patients and families on the ward. The health-care team needs to attend to the needs of the bereaved as well as those of patients not involved!

Table 24.3 Tenets of religions that have implications for the care of patients

Meaning: Mindful life review – a verbal or written review of his or her biography by a patient, striving to break repetitous thinking, to get close to an understanding of life's meaning and to be reconciled with it.

Connectedness: Participation in rituals (celebration of crises and transitions, using the exacting symbols familiar to all participants).

Singing, praying or being silent together all reconnect an existentially isolated person with something beyond the present suffering and isolation.

Organizing good-byes, preparing some kind of legacy are ways to reaffirm and bring to a closure existing relationships.

Forgiveness and acceptance: Understanding the universality of sin, regret and guilt can be fostered by reading sacred writings, selected poetry, etc.

Caregivers can manifest the possibility of forgiveness only by the way they accept the patient.

Loved ones who cannot forgive the dying person should be encouraged to promise that forgiveness will take place, even though posthumously ('stored' forgiveness, TM Smeding).

Hope: The direct question 'What do you hope for at this point in your life?' triggers reflection that goes beyond issues of tumor size.

A 'stepladder of hope' may go from cure to healing via hopes for symptom control, for loved ones, for reconciliation.

Transcendence: 'Man is never helped in his suffering by what he thinks of himself; only suprahuman, revealed truth lifts him out of his distress' (CG Jung).

The experience of being overwhelmed by something beyond his suffering can happen to anyone. But it cannot be made – only facilitated.

Signpost

Several studies have shown better outcomes in cancer patients practicing a religion.

Acknowledgments

I thank Dr Ruthmarijke Smeding and the Rev. Michael Wright, Senior Research Fellow at the International Observatory on End of Life Care, Lancaster University, UK, for valuable help.

Further reading

Frankl V: Man's Search for Meaning, 3rd edn. New York: Washington Square Press,1984.

George RJ (ed): Evaluation and Treatment of Chronic Pain in the Native American Patient. ACOFF CME Supplement November 2004. www.acofp.org/member_publications/1104_Supplement.pdf#search='Ma ugen%20SPIRITual%20History'

Int J Palliat Nurs 1997; 3(1) and 1998, 4(4): Special issues on spiritual cases.

Kearney M: Mortally Wounded: Stories of Soul Pain, Death and Healing. Dublin: Marino, 1996.

O'Neill B, Fallon M. ABC of palliative care. Principles of palliative care and pain control. BMJ 1997; 315: 801–4.

Puchalski CM: Spirituality and end-of-life care: a time for listening and caring. J Palliat Med 2002; 5: 289–94.

Speck P: Spiritual/religious issues in care of the dying. In: Ellershaw J Wilkinson S (eds), Care of the Dying – A Pathway to Excellence. Oxford: Oxford University Press, 2003.

Weiher E: Mehr als Begleiten – Ein neues Profil für die Seelsorge im Raum von Medizin und Pflege. Mainz: Grünewald, 1999.

Wright M: www.lancs.ac.uk/fss/ihr/staff/michaelwright.htm

Appendix 1
Edmonton Symptom Assessment System (ESAS)

Purpose of the ESAS

This tool is designed to assist in the assessment of nine symptoms common in cancer patients: pain, tiredness, nausea, depression, anxiety, drowsiness, appetite, wellbeing and shortness of breath, (there is also a line labelled "Other Problem"). The severity **at the time of assessment** of each symptom is rated from 0 to 10 on a numerical scale, 0 meaning that the symptom is absent and 10 that it is of the worst possible severity. The patient and family should be taught how to complete the scales. It is the <u>patient's opinion</u> on the severity of the symptoms that is the "gold standard" for symptom assessment.

The ESAS provides a clinical profile of symptom severity over time. It provides a context within which symptoms can begin to be understood. However, it is not a complete symptom assessment itself. For good symptom management to be attained the ESAS must be used as just one part of a holistic clinical assessment.

How to do the ESAS

| No pain | 0 1 2 3 4 5 6 7 8 9 10 | Worse possible pain |

The circled number is then transcribed onto the symptom assessment graph (see " ESAS Graph") below.

Synonyms for words that may be difficult for some patients to comprehend include the following:

Depression	– blue or sad
Anxiety	– nervousness or restlessness
Tiredness	– decreased energy level (but not necessarily sleepy)
Drowsiness	– sleepiness
Wellbeing	– overall comfort, both physical and otherwise; truthfully answering the question, "How are you?"

When to do the ESAS

a) In palliative home care, it is good practice to complete and graph the ESAS during each telephone or personal contact. If symptoms are in good control, and there are no predominant psychosocial issues, the ESAS can be completed weekly for patients in the home. In hospice and tertiary palliative care units the ESAS should be completed daily. In other settings the palliative consultants will utilize this tool in their assessment on each visit.

b) If the patient's symptoms are not in good control, daily assessments need to be done in person by the attending health professionals until the symptoms are well-controlled (see "d" below).

c) If symptom management is not attained, or consultation about possible care options is needed, patient assessments by Palliative Care Consultants are available (**attending physician must agree**). Consultative discussions not requiring in-person assessments are available from Palliative Care Consultants upon request.

d) If, after all therapeutic options have been exhausted and consensus is reached that a symptom cannot be further improved, visits and assessments can return to their normal pattern for that patient.

Who should do the ESAS

Ideally, patients fill out their own ESAS. However, if the patient is cognitively impaired or for other reasons cannot independently do the ESAS, then it is completed with the assistance of a caregiver (a family member, friend, or health professional closely involved in the patient's care). If the patient cannot participate in the symptom assessment, or refuses to do so, the ESAS is completed by the caregiver alone.

Note: when the ESAS is completed by the caregiver alone the subjective symptom scales are not done (i.e. tiredness, depression, anxiety, and wellbeing are left blank) and the caregiver assesses the remaining symptoms as objectively as possible, i.e. pain is assessed on the basis of a knowledge of pain behaviors, appetite is interpreted as the absence or presence of eating, nausea as the absence or presence of retching or vomiting, and shortness of breath as laboured or accelerated respirations that appears to be causing distress for the patient.

When a patient is irreversibly cognitively impaired and cannot participate in doing the ESAS, the caregiver continues to complete the ESAS as outlined

<u>above</u> and the Edmonton Comfort Assessment FORM (ECAF) may also be used (see ECAF guidelines).

The method in which the ESAS was completed must be indicated in the space provided at the bottom of the ESAS Numerical Scale and the ESAS Graph as follows:

Bottom of ESAS Numerical Scale

Completed by (*check one*)

Patient   ❏
Caregiver   ❏
Caregiver-assisted ❏

Bottom of ESAS Graph

Completed by ❏❏❏❏❏❏   Insert appropriate letter from key in date
                        column (date indicated at the top of form)

Key:

P = Patient   ❏
C = Caregiver   ❏
A = Caregiver-assisted ❏

Where to document the ESAS

The ESAS is always done on the ESAS Numerical Scale and the results _later transferred_ to the ESAS Graph. Graphing symptom severity directly onto the ESAS Graph without the use of the numerical scale is not a valid use of the ESAS nor a reliable method of symptom assessment (attention to the graphed historical trend may affect the current scores and so undermine one of the main purposes of the ESAS, i.e. to assess the <u>current</u> symptom profile as accurately as possible).

Other information about the ESAS

The ESAS Graph also contains space to add the patient's Mini-Mental Status Exam score. The "normal" box refers to the normal range for the patient, based on age and education level (see Instructions for MMSE). As well, a space for the Palliative Performance Scale (PPS) is included. The ESAS is available in other languages and also in faces for those patients who do not read.

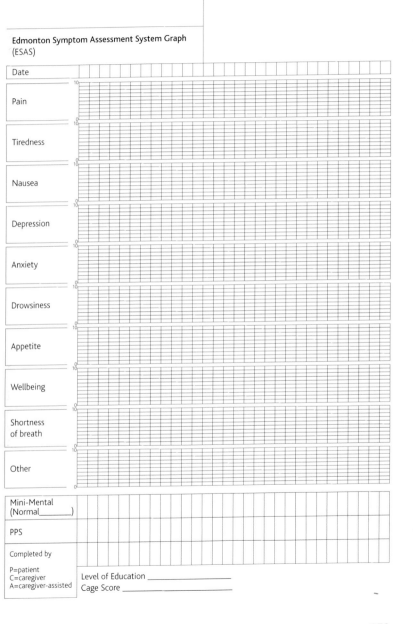

Edmonton Symptom Assessment System Graph (ESAS)

Date																							

Pain 10–0

Tiredness 10–0

Nausea 10–0

Depression 10–0

Anxiety 10–0

Drowsiness 10–0

Appetite 10–0

Wellbeing 10–0

Shortness of breath 10–0

Other 10–0

Mini-Mental (Normal_____)																							
PPS																							
Completed by																							

P=patient
C=caregiver
A=caregiver-assisted

Level of Education _____
Cage Score _____

Edmonton Symptom Assessment System:
Numerical Scale
Regional Palliative Care Program

Please circle the number that best describes:

No pain	0 1 2 3 4 5 6 7 8 9 10	Worst possible pain
Not tired	0 1 2 3 4 5 6 7 8 9 10	Worst possible tiredness
Not nauseated	0 1 2 3 4 5 6 7 8 9 10	Worst possible nausea
Not depressed	0 1 2 3 4 5 6 7 8 9 10	Worst possible depression
Not anxious	0 1 2 3 4 5 6 7 8 9 10	Worst possible anxiety
Not drowsy	0 1 2 3 4 5 6 7 8 9 10	Worst possible drowsiness
Best appetite	0 1 2 3 4 5 6 7 8 9 10	Worst possible appetite
Best feeling of wellbeing	0 1 2 3 4 5 6 7 8 9 10	Worst possible feeling of wellbeing
No shortness of breath	0 1 2 3 4 5 6 7 8 9 10	Worst possible shortness of breath
Other problem	0 1 2 3 4 5 6 7 8 9 10	

Patient's Name _____

Date _____ Time _____

Complete by (*check one*)

☐ Patient
☐ Caregiver
☐ Caregiver assisted

Please mark on these pictures where it is you hurt.

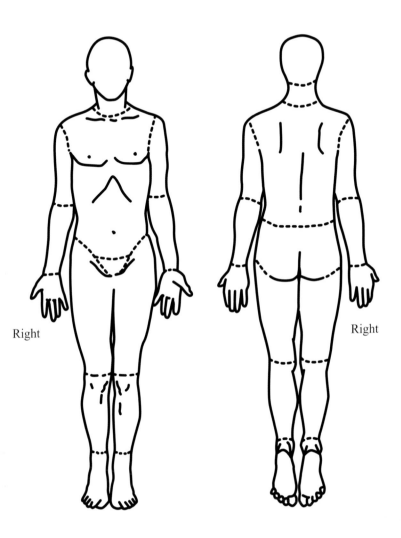

Right

Right

Appendix 2
ESMO policy on supportive and palliative care

Policy 1: The role of the oncologist in the provision of supportive and palliative care

The medical oncologist must be skilled in supportive and palliative care of patients with cancer and in end-of-life care. Consequently, specific training in these skills must be a part of the core curriculum of all accredited training programs.

The delivery of supportive and palliative care to cancer patients requires an appropriate medical nursing and paramedical infrastructure to address the special needs of these patients and their families. It is the responsibility of medical oncologists to assess and evaluate physical and psychological symptoms of patients under their care and to ensure that these problems are adequately addressed.

The delivery of high-quality supportive and palliative care requires cooperation and coordination with physicians from other disciplines (e.g. radiotherapy, surgery, rehabilitation, psycho-oncology, pain medicine and anesthesiology and palliative medicine), as well as with paramedical clinicians (nursing, social work, psychology, physical and occupational therapy, chaplains, and others).

Regarding end-of-life care for cancer patients, ESMO endorses the Core Principles for End-of-Life Care. Care at the end of life should:

- respect the dignity of both the patient and caregivers
- be sensitive to and respectful of the patient's and family's wishes
- use the most appropriate measures that are consistent with patient choices
- make alleviation of pain and other physical symptoms a high priority
- recognize that good care for the dying person requires expert medical care but also entails services that are family- and community-based in order to address, for example, psychological, social and spiritual/religious problems

- offer continuity (patients should be able to continue to be cared for, if so desired, by their primary care and medical oncology providers)
- advocate access to therapies that can reasonably be expected to improve patients' quality of life, and ensure that patients who choose alternative or nontraditional treatments are not abandoned
- provide access to palliative care and hospice care
- respect the patient's right to refuse treatment, as expressed by the patient or an authorized surrogate
- respect the physician's professional responsibility to discontinue some treatments when appropriate, with consideration for both patient and family preferences
- promote clinical and evidence-based research on providing care at the end of life.

Policy 2: ESMO policy regarding supportive and palliative care training for medical oncologists

Medical oncologists must be skilled in the supportive and palliative care of patients with advanced cancer. Consequently, specific training in these skills must be part of the curriculum of all accredited training programs.

Nine core skills must be incorporated:

1. *Oncological management of advanced cancer*
   Medical oncologists must be expert in the appropriate use of antitumor therapies as palliative techniques when cure is no longer possible. This includes specific familiarity with key concepts of patient benefit, quality of life and risk–benefit analysis.

2. *Communication with patients and family members*
   The medical oncologist must be skilled in effective and compassionate communication with cancer patients and their families. Specific skills include explaining diagnosis and treatment options, disclosure of diagnoses, explaining issues relating to prognosis, explaining the potential risks and benefits of treatment options, counseling skills to facilitate effective and informed decision making, explaining the role of palliative care, and care of distressed family members (fear, anticipatory grief, bereavement care and the convening of family meetings).

3. *Management of complications of cancer*
   Medical oncologists must be expert in the evaluation and management of the complications of cancer, including bone metastases, central nervous system metastases (brain and leptomeningeal metastases), neurological

dysfunction (primary, metastatic, paraneoplastic and iatrogenic), liver metastases and biliary obstruction, malignant effusions (pleural, peritoneal and pericardial), obstruction of hollow viscera (esophagus, airways, gastric outlet, small and large bowel, and ureters), metabolic consequences of cancer, anorexia and cachexia, and hematological consequences (anemia, neutropenia, thrombocytopenia, clotting diathesis and sexual dysfunction).

4. *Evaluation and management of physical symptoms of cancer and cancer treatment*

Medical oncologists must be expert in the evaluation and management of the common physical symptoms of advanced cancer, including pain, dyspnea and cough, fatigue, nausea and vomiting, constipation, diarrhea, insomnia, and itch.

5. *Evaluation and management of psychological and existential symptoms of cancer*

Medical oncologists must be familiar with the evaluation and management of the common psychological and existential symptoms of cancer, including anxiety, depression, delirium, suicidal desire or desire for death, death anxiety, and anticipatory grief.

6. *Interdisciplinary care*

Medical oncologists must be familiar with the roles of other professions in the care of patients with cancer and with community resources to support the care of these patients.

7. *Palliative care research*

Medical oncologists must be familiar with research methodologies that are applicable to patients with cancer, including quality-of-life research, pain measurement and research, measurement of other physical and psychological symptoms (dyspnea, fatigue, nausea and vomiting, depression and anxiety, and desire for death), needs evaluation, decision-making research, and palliative care audit.

8. *Ethical issues in the management of patients with cancer*

Medical oncologists must be familiar with common ethical problems that arise in the management of advanced cancer and with ethical principles that assist in resolving these problems: ethical issues related to disclosure of diagnosis and prognosis; ethical issues in decision making (paternalism, autonomy and informed consent); and the right to adequate relief of physical and psychological symptoms and its implications; ethical issues at the end of life (sedation for refractory symptoms, hydration and nutrition at the end of life, daunorubicin, and the use of invasive palliative approaches, such as nephrostomy or dialysis); forgoing treatment; and issues related to euthanasia and assisted suicide.

9. *Preventing burnout*

The medical oncologist must be familiar with the symptoms of burnout, the factors that contribute to burnout and strategies to prevent its development. Different levels of competence are expected for different core skills: 'expert' refers to a high level of academic and practical knowledge; 'skilled' refers to effective clinical competence; and 'familiar' refers to familiarity with core concepts, sufficient for adequately evaluating the patient, initiating basic therapy and communicating with clinical experts.

At the completion of training, graduates should be expert in the oncological management of advanced cancer, the management of complications of cancer, and the evaluation and management of physical symptoms of cancer and cancer treatment. They should be skilled in communication with patients and family members, and they should be familiar with the evaluation and management of psychological and existential symptoms of cancer, the interdisciplinary care of patients who have advanced cancer, palliative care research, ethical issues in the management of patients with cancer, and prevention of burnout.

Policy 3: ESMO policy regarding minimum standards for the provision of supportive and palliative care by cancer centers

Since most cancer patients receive their cancer care in dedicated clinics or hospitals, it is imperative that these facilities provide an adequate supportive and palliative care infrastructure as part of the overall service. Key tasks of supportive and palliative care provision in the cancer center include the screening of cancer patients to identify those who have specific needs, and the provision of real-time supportive and palliative care interventions as part of routine cancer care.

The minimum requirements of palliative care in the cancer center are as follows:

■ Cancer patients (especially those who have advanced cancer) receiving active therapy in cancer centers should be routinely assessed for the presence and severity of physical and psychological symptoms and for the adequacy of social supports.

- When inadequately controlled symptoms are identified, they must be evaluated and treated with the appropriate urgency, depending on the nature and severity of the problem.
- The cancer center must provide skilled emergency care for inadequately relieved physical and psychological symptoms.
- Cancer centers must maintain a program of palliative and supportive care for patients with advanced cancer who no longer derive any benefit from antitumor interventions.
- Cancer centers should incorporate social work and psychological care into routine care.
- When patients require inpatient end-of-life care, the cancer center staff should either provide the needed inpatient care or arrange adequate care in an appropriate hospice or palliative care service.

Index